5 SQUARE

LOW-CARB MEALS

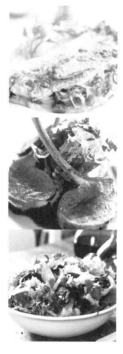

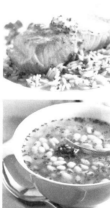

5 SQUARE

LOW-CARB MEALS

THE 20-DAY MAKEOVER PLAN WITH DELICIOUS RECIPES

FOR FAST, HEALTHY WEIGHT LOSS AND HIGH ENERGY

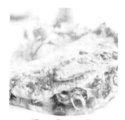

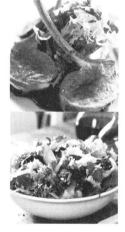

M O N I C A   L Y N N

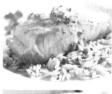

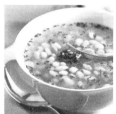

1⊕ ReganBooks
Celebrating Ten Bestselling Years
An Imprint of HarperCollins*Publishers*

5 SQUARE LOW-CARB MEALS. Copyright © 2004 by Monica Lynn. All rights reserved. Printed in the United States of America. No part of this book may be used or reproduced in any manner whatsoever without written permission except in the case of brief quotations embodied in critical articles and reviews. For information address HarperCollins Publishers Inc., 10 East 53rd Street, New York, NY 10022.

HarperCollins books may be purchased for educational, business, or sales promotional use. For information please write: Special Markets Department, HarperCollins Publishers Inc., 10 East 53rd Street, New York, NY 10022.

FIRST EDITION

Designed by Richard Oriolo

Printed on acid-free paper

Library of Congress Cataloging-in-Publication Data has been applied for.

ISBN 0-06-058999-X
04 05 06 07 08 WBC/RRD 10 9 8 7 6 5 4 3 2 1

This book is dedicated to Linda Carpenito Ciaramella—I miss you!

ACKNOWLEDGMENTS

I want to thank the following people for all their help and support:

To Judith Regan for being an inspiration; you are truly an amazing woman. Your staff and their expertise helped me throughout this process and I am so grateful for everyone's help, from my editor, the "sweet girl next door," Aliza Fogelson, to my beautiful and talented new friend and art director Michelle Ishay.

To the Barshop family, for putting my head back into business mode. You and your children mean so much to me and continue to motivate me every step of the way.

To Shari Aaron, my muse. You will never know how grateful I am for your support and guidance.

To Jim Paretti, for believing in me, 5 squares, and *the show that will be*, I promise.

To Gary Blum and the Laurus Group, for continuously helping me put 5 squares on the map—you guys are the best!

To Tim DeBaets and his talented team, thank you for looking out for me.

To my own "can't-live-without her, fabulous right hand," Jacklyn Rodriguez. Thank you for your loyalty and for putting up with me—never an easy task!

To Ed Papick, my unofficial business consultant and dear friend. You are a genius and I am so proud of you and your accomplishments. You will rule, my friend!

To Danny Savino, Dianna Calderon, and Anthony Spina, thank you for saving my life.

To Page Falkinburg, a.k.a. Diamond Dallas Page, who has mastered the art of self-promotion. I am so proud of you.

To Laura Vecchio, for being such a great friend and loyal employee.

To all my clients, I thank you for your continued support and loyalty. Without you, none of this would be possible. A very special thanks to my Darien ladies, keep talking! Gail Reynolds, you put me on the map in Darien and you will never believe how important you were in making 5 squares a success. Amy Paul, my very first customer—always cutting edge—you are gorgeous!

To Peter Berley, I thank you for your never-ending talent and patience. Re-writing these recipes was not an easy task. You rose to the occasion!

To my family, I thank God every day for you. Mom, you are my best friend and I love you for letting me call you seven times a day. No one ever said raising me was easy: You did a great job, if I may say so myself. A special hug to my nieces Isabella, Brianna, Sofia, and my nephew Brett; you bring such joy to my life. I love every minute of watching you grow.

CONTENTS

STAYING ON TRACK: BEYOND THE 5 SQUARE MEAL

5 SQUARE

LOW-CARB MEALS

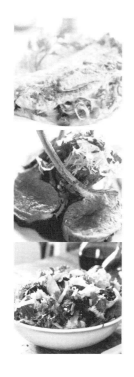

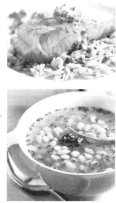

Food, food, food . . . everything in my life was focused around that four-letter word. I was raised in a family plagued by obesity, and growing up in the restaurant business was like living on Temptation Island. My parents were of no help; my father—who at times ballooned to over 350 pounds—was the master of the den. He brought home his offerings and cooked them up for his cubs—wonderful sauces over pasta like Fettuccine Alfredo, homemade pizzas, and delicious empanadas (a staple from Argentina where he was born and raised). My mother, with her most famous dish of all, mayonnaise fried chicken and creamed mashed potatoes, could entice even the most health-conscious individual into grabbing another drumstick.

When I was 12, my father opened his first restaurant: Scampi's Italian Seafood House in North Miami Beach. It was a great place to grow up: I would pop a quarter into the jukebox, lather up the garlic bread, and serve it to the grateful patrons while belting out Barbra Streisand tunes. The food was amazing: fresh clams shucked to order, homemade pastas, and their signature shrimp scampi. Of course, I assumed the clientele came to hear my rendition of "You Don't Bring Me Flowers," but when I got demoted to dishwasher, business still boomed.

Our next restaurant during my youth was best known for its Belgian waffles and damn-good homemade ice cream: who could resist? My father was a culinary genius and his creativity always amazed me; he could take the simplest of ingredients and orchestrate culinary delights.

Food was always a major event in my family and the effects began to be apparent. By 1997, my father was diagnosed as a Type II diabetic and my entire family was plagued with weight issues. It hit me when I was approaching my thirties. I thought I was blessed with a superhuman metabolism. As my siblings grew into the obese category, my weight gain was more insidious.

Slowly, my clothing began to "shrink," and quite frankly, my waist began to expand. Instead of fooling myself that the washing machine repairman would fix this problem, I decided it was time to hit the gym. I became the aerobic queen, spinning, kickboxing, jumping up and down until my shins ached. But I noticed that my clothes were still getting tighter, and I was famished all the time. I remember sitting on top of the kitchen counter inhaling so-called "diet foods" like "low-fat" cookies at midnight—or eating a whole pint of "fat-free" ice cream . . . Does this sound familiar?

The more I ate, the hungrier I got. The more I worked out, the hungrier I got. The more I stressed out over it . . . well, you get the picture. My problems with my eating habits became far too great for me to handle myself (or so I thought). I felt I needed to seek "professional help." But I didn't need a therapist for counseling; I needed to go on a *diet!* Every day, millions of people go on diets. They lose a few pounds and feel as if they are "home free," only to find the pounds returning when they resort back to regular eating habits. *Why is this?* As you probably know, and as I learned the hard way, the answer is that very few *diets* work. We've learned that anyone can lose weight drinking a few shakes all day, or eating frozen, overprocessed concoctions from the supermarket—but we still face the question: what happens when you *stop?* There are many pills and potions out there for a quick fix, but most of us end up feeling worse than we did before we started our quests to lose weight.

I tried every diet from starvation to frozen meals, shakes, and diet pills, even a cabbage soup diet. I noticed that I'd drop a few pounds that would creep back up on me the minute I returned to my normal eating habits. I read numerous diet books and fitness magazines and came to the realization that I needed to change my whole way of thinking.

I spent a lot of evenings at the gym—my personal life was not even half as exciting as watching those beautiful buff men and women bench press and do leg lifts. How did they do it? I often wondered. How did they stay so lean and full of energy? Better-than-average genetics? I used to watch the bodybuilders pump iron and then sit down and pull out a baggie or Tupperware full of food and consume it right there at the gym. I finally got up the nerve to venture over to one of them and literally begged him for his secret. *"What is it that you do to stay so lean, and why are you always eating?"* I asked. *"Eat more, eat clean,"* he said. "Eat more, eat clean?" I repeated. He smiled and walked away to continue with his impressive regimen. I watched him—who wouldn't have? And as I turned over his response in my mind, I thought I might be on to something.

I took the next couple of weeks to pore over books, magazines, and videos, anything I could read or watch to learn more about members of the fitness world and their eating habits.

I consulted a nutritionist, a cardiologist, even a bariatric specialist, because I wanted to make the right personal lifestyle changes. I learned so much—but more exciting than learning was executing. I began creating shopping lists and menus, and planned my eating times by actually making an appointment in my date book—just as I would for an official meeting or other commitment. (It really works to help keep you on a consistent schedule!) The key, I learned, was to *"Eat more"*—at least five times a day to keep your metabolism running at its maximum performance level, and *"Eat clean"*—eliminate all empty calories (wheat, dairy, and most important, sugar), and *Plan ahead*—the time that you eat and what you are eating should be planned in advance.

I consulted my doctors and got their blessing. They reviewed the parameters and assured me that not only was the plan healthy, but balanced and sensible, as well. Thanks to my culinary upbringing, I became the master of healthy meals—cooking, preparing, and packaging my own food to consume throughout the day. At the time, I was the owner of a popular hair and nail salon and my clients watched me shrink down in size—while I popped out of my seat to eat delicious healthy meals every three hours! I had never felt better! My employees and clients all watched in awe as my weight dropped, and they wanted to know what my secret was. "It's no secret," I said. *"Eat more, eat clean!"*

Before long, I was cooking for them, too. Within six weeks, I had lost 14 pounds, 30 percent of my body fat, felt better than I had in years, changed my lifestyle, sold my salon, and started a new business, helping others achieve their weight loss and lifestyle goals.

I devised a way not only to prepare meals for others, but to deliver them fresh to their homes every day. My delivery service, 5 squares™, has successfully assisted thousands of people, and continues to do so every day. I was inspired by seeing the phenomenal difference that eating 5 "squares"—5 healthy, balanced meals—each day has made in my clients' lives, and I decided to bring the basic principles of the 5 squares lifestyle to readers beyond the scope of my delivery service. That's why I created the 5 Square Meal Makeover Plan, a twenty-day program based on the same ideas as my 5 squares business, but adapted so that you'll have all the recipes and tips you need to follow the plan at home. Because my delivery service and this book follow the same outline, I interchangeably refer to the 5 squares plan and the 5 Square Meal Makeover Plan throughout the book.

The plan is simple and with this book you can easily change your weight, your body image, and your life! *Eat more, eat clean;* eliminate refined sugars and wheat, stay away from dairy, and eat all day long! I knew it was time to share my secret and I have mapped out a program that can easily be adapted into any situation. So read on, and make the healthy lifestyle change you have thought about for years. Five square meals a day = more digestion = more efficiency in burning calories = more weight loss.

GETTING STARTED

MAINTAINING WEIGHT

The first step in making the change is to evaluate what your caloric needs are. For adult men and women, many doctors use the following calculation method:

If you live a largely sedentary lifestyle—meaning you do not do any extra physical activity other than your normal daily routine—caloric needs are generally 13 times your body weight (in pounds). This is to *maintain* your current weight; for example, if you want to *maintain* a current weight of 150 pounds, you should be eating 1950 calories per day (13 times 150).

For those with a moderately active lifestyle—you go to the gym three times per week or you power walk or exercise frequently (three or more times per week)—your caloric needs are 15 times weight. So if you weigh 150 pounds, you should be eating around 2250 calories per day just to *maintain* your current weight.

Those with a strenuous lifestyle (very active, high metabolism) will require approximately 20 times weight, which would be 3000 calories a day if you weigh 150 pounds.

I have included this chart with examples of weights and the amount of calories it takes to *sustain* your current weight:

CALORIES PER DAY NECESSARY TO MAINTAIN WEIGHT

WEIGHT IN POUNDS	SEDENTARY	MODERATE	ACTIVE
130	1690	1950	2600
135	1755	2025	2700
140	1820	2100	2800
145	1885	2175	2900
150	1950	2250	3000
155	2015	2325	3100
160	2080	2400	3200
165	2145	2475	3300
170	2210	2550	3400
175	2275	2625	3500
180	2340	2700	3600
185	2405	2775	3700
190	2470	2850	3800
195	2535	2925	3900
200	2600	3000	4000
210	2730	3150	4200
220	2860	3300	4400
230	2990	3450	4600
240	3120	3600	4800
250	3250	3750	5000
260	3380	3900	5200
270	3510	4050	5400
280	3640	4200	5600
290	3770	4350	5800
300	3900	4500	6000
310	4030	4650	6200
320	4160	4800	6400
330	4290	4950	6600
340	4420	5100	6800
350	4550	5250	7000
360	4680	5400	7200

LOSING WEIGHT

For weight loss, a reduction of approximately 500 calories per day should result in an average weight loss of approximately 1 pound per week.

What does this mean? If you decrease your intake by just 500 calories per day, you can expect to lose about 4 pounds per month. Remember, as your weight goes down, the amount of calories you will need to consume decreases as well.

One of the key elements to success on the 5 Square Meal Makeover Plan is to reduce your consumption of sugar and wheat. Many of us have difficulty losing weight because of our high consumption of sugar—often, more than we know.

ARE YOU ADDICTED TO SUGAR? A SIMPLE QUIZ

The following quiz will help you determine how important refined sugars are in your life. By "refined" I mean sugar that is processed in any way by anything, human or insect (bees), as opposed to "natural" sugar, which is found in fruits and vegetables. Refined sugars include sucrose, honey, fructose, glucose, dextrose, levulose, maltose, raw sugar, brown sugar, maple sugar, barley malt, rice syrup, and corn sweeteners. These are all considered "simple" sugars because they are absorbed into the bloodstream quickly and digested rapidly. They are typically found in junk foods such as doughnuts and candy bars but can also be found in condiments, salad dressings, "fat-free" products, and canned fruit.

Answer the following questions as truthfully as possible.

True or False:

I eat some form of refined sugar every day. _____

I often have cravings for chocolate, peanut butter, alcohol, or sugar. _____

I sometimes hide sweets around my home to eat at a later time. _____

I find that it is difficult to stop eating candy after one piece,
or one bite of dessert. _____

I cannot have candy in my home and not eat it. _____

I want something sweet after every meal. _____

I drink coffee and eat a sweet breakfast every day. _____

I drink sweetened beverages every day. _____

If you answered "true" to more than three of these statements, you are more than likely addicted to sugar. You crave sugar and probably eat it frequently. I could explain the biological causes behind this, and I could give you hundreds of reasons why not to eat sugar, but that's not the focus of this book. The bottom line is that you can stop the cycle now. . . . *5 Square Low-Carb Meals* will help. You will feel a difference in just 3 days! You will feel more energy and less bloating. And soon, the pounds will come off and you'll be feeling better than ever!

SUGAR WEARS MANY MASKS

One of the problems with regulating consumption of sugars is being able to identify certain foods with "hidden" sugars. Did you know?

- Some salt contains sugar.

- Sugar is often added to canned fruits.

- Alcoholic beverages such as wine and beer contain sugar. Champagne and cordials have an even higher amount of sugar.

- Bouillon cubes generally contain sugar. Sugar is often used in the processing of luncheon meats and canned meats.

- Poultry is often injected with a honey solution prior to being sold to fast-food restaurants.

- Commercial ketchups are loaded with sugar (almost 50 percent of the calories are from sugar).

- A 10-ounce glass of orange juice contains the juice of approximately 8 large oranges, which is equivalent to nine teaspoons of sugar.

Take note: Refined sugar is 99.5 percent *pure calories*—no vitamins, no minerals, and no proteins, just simply carbohydrates. According to statistics, the average person eats over 10 pounds of sugar each month, which is nearly 4½ cups of sugar per week. On the 5 Square Meal Makeover Plan, you'll be cutting down on your sugar intake and instead eating healthier, more nutritious foods.

EXERCISE

Exercise is essential in any weight-loss program. The truth of the matter is that 70 percent of Americans just don't do it. Our sedentary lifestyles figure largely in why we are the fattest nation in the world. Burning calories and building lean muscle mass through exercise speeds weight loss and improves our health and general feeling of well-being.

Examples of exercise and the calories we expend:

CALORIES BURNED PER 1 HOUR OF ACTIVITY

ACTIVITY	130 LBS	155 LBS	190 LBS
Aerobics, general	354	422	518
Aerobics, high impact	413	493	604
Aerobics, low impact	295	352	431
Baseball, competitive	531	633	776
Baseball, playing catch	148	176	216
Backpacking	413	493	604
Basketball, game	472	563	690
Basketball, shooting baskets	266	317	388
Bicycling <10 mph	236	281	345
Bicycling 10–12 mph	354	422	518
Bicycling 12–14 mph	472	563	690
Bicycling, stationary, general	295	352	431
Bicycling, stationary, vigorous	738	880	1078
Bowling	177	211	259
Boxing, punching bag	354	422	518
Child care, general	207	246	302
Circuit training, general	472	563	690
Cleaning, general house	207	246	302
Cooking, food preparation	148	176	216
Dancing, ballroom	177	211	259

ACTIVITY	130 LBS	155 LBS	190 LBS
Dancing, general	266	317	388
Fishing, general	236	281	345
Football, competitive	531	633	776
Football, playing catch	148	176	216
Frisbee	177	211	259
Gardening	295	352	431
Golf, general	236	281	345
Golf, miniature or driving range	177	211	259
Handball, general	708	844	1035
Hiking, cross country	354	422	518
Hockey, field	472	563	690
Hockey, ice	472	563	690
Horseback riding, general	236	281	345
Hunting, general	295	352	431
Jogging	413	493	604
Judo/Karate	590	704	863
Kayaking	295	352	431
Marching band	236	281	345
Mowing lawn	325	387	474
Paddleboat	236	281	345
Painting/Wallpapering	266	317	388
Playing with child, walking/running	236	281	345
Pushing or pulling stroller	148	176	216
Racquetball, competitive	590	704	863
Racquetball, general	413	493	604
Raking lawn	236	281	345
Rock climbing, ascending	649	774	949
Rock climbing, rappelling	472	563	690
Rope jumping, general	590	704	863
Rowing, stationary, moderate effort	413	493	604
Running 5 mph	472	563	690
Running in place (or StairMaster)	472	563	690
Running, up stairs	885	1056	1294
Running 10 mph	944	1126	1380
Sailing	177	211	259

ACTIVITY	130 LBS	155 LBS	190 LBS
Sailing, competitive	295	352	431
Skiing, cross country, moderate	472	563	690
Skiing, downhill, moderate	354	422	518
Skiing, water	354	422	518
Sledding	413	493	604
Snorkeling	295	352	431
Snowmobiling	207	246	302
Snow shoeing	472	563	690
Soccer, casual	413	493	604
Soccer, competitive	590	704	863
Softball	295	352	431
Stair-treadmill	354	422	518
Stretching/yoga	236	281	345
Surfing	177	211	259
Swimming laps	472	563	690
Table tennis/ping pong	236	281	345
Tennis, doubles	354	422	518
Tennis, general	413	493	604
Volleyball, beach	472	563	690
Volleyball, competitive, gymnasium	236	281	345
Walking, slow pace	148	176	216
Walking, treadmill at 4 mph	236	281	345
Walking, uphill	354	422	518
Walking, very briskly/power walk	236	281	345
Walking dog	207	246	302
Weightlifting, light	177	211	259
Weightlifting, vigorous	354	422	518
Whitewater rafting	295	352	431

If you have not exercised in a long time, it is best to start off slowly. Begin the first week with an activity for fifteen minutes, three times during the week. You'll want to choose an exercise that maximizes your caloric burn such as power walking. Add fifteen minutes to your daily routine every two weeks until you have reached an hour of activity, three times during the week or strive for a minimum of 700 calories burned per week. You should consult your doctor before beginning any exercise program.

HOW THE **5 SQUARE** MEAL MAKEOVER PLAN WORKS

WHAT TO EAT

The plan is based on eating five balanced meals, or "squares" each day. The meals you will eat will be made up of three categories: proteins, starches (starchy carbohydrates), and vegetables (fibrous carbohydrates).

GROUP A (PROTEINS)	AMOUNT
Chicken, boneless, skinless white meat	6 ounces, precooked
Turkey breast, boneless, skinless white meat	6 ounces, precooked
Turkey, ground, 98 percent fat-free	6 ounces, precooked
Fish, salmon (limit to two times per week)	4 ounces, precooked
Fish, white	6 ounces, precooked
Shrimp/scallops/lobster	4 ounces, precooked
Beef/veal/pork, lean cuts (limit to two times per week)	4 ounces, precooked
Egg whites	4 to 6

In addition to being a good source of protein for vegetarians and vegans, *tofu* can be a great substitute in some of the recipes in this book, especially in place of chicken or turkey. A serving size of tofu is 1 cup, or about 8 ounces.

Because they are rich in fiber, *beans* are also a good option as a source of protein. On the down side, they are high in carbohydrates, so you'll want to be sure to balance meals that contain beans with some of the previously mentioned lean, lower-carb protein sources. It's best not to add additional starch to meals which contain beans. A serving size of most types of beans is about 1 cup.

GROUP B (STARCHES)	AMOUNT
Potato, sweet or white	4 ounces, cooked
Rice, preferably brown	½ cup, cooked
Barley	½ cup, cooked
Spelt bread	1 slice
Oatmeal	½ cup, precooked
Corn (limit to one time per week)	½ cup/2 mini ears

GROUP C (VEGETABLES)	AMOUNT
Any leafy green vegetable	minimum ½ cup cooked
Any fibrous vegetable (see list below)	minimum ½ cup cooked

Choose mostly leafy green vegetables and limit your intake of carrots to twice per week.

Some examples of great fibrous vegetables are:

Asparagus	Eggplant	Onions
Broccoli	Escarole	Peppers
Broccoli rabe	Kale	Salad mixes, baby greens
Cauliflower	Leeks	Spinach
Cucumbers	Mushrooms	Zucchini

The following vegetables should be used in moderation (no more than ½ cup cooked or 4 ounces per serving), as they are rather starchy:

| Carrots | Turnips |
| Peas | Water chestnuts |

As you will see, each meal, or what I call throughout the book a "square," is composed of a specific proportion of protein, starch, and vegetable. This has been calculated for you in the sample menus and recipes.

SQUARE #1	protein (A) + starch (B) + vegetable (C)
SQUARE #2	protein (A) + vegetable (C)
SQUARE #3	protein (A) + starch (B) + vegetable (C)
SQUARE #4	protein (A) + vegetable (C)
SQUARE #5	protein (A) + starch (B) + vegetable (C)

For ease of use during the plan, we've classified all the recipes into one of these 5 squares based on the proportions above. However, you can experiment with mixing and matching the meals in the recipe pages. For example, because Square #2 and Square #4 contain the same proportions of protein and vegetable, you can exchange the recipe choices in Square #2 (pages 61–83), your mid-morning snack, with those from Square #4 (pages 123–144), your midday snack. You can do the same with lunch, Square #3 (pages 87–119), and dinner, Square #5 (pages 147–180), as they contain approximately the same proportions of protein, vegetable, and starch.

For example, using the suggested sample menu on page 24, you might decide to eat the Chicken, Barley, and Vegetable Soup in the afternoon, and the Barbecued Grilled Chicken with Sweet and Sour Cucumbers as your mid-afternoon snack. Similarly, you might prefer to eat Stuffed Eggplant with Mashed Sweet Potatoes as your dinner, and to eat Oatmeal-Almond-Crusted Flounder with Spicy Sautéed String Beans and Lemon Zest for your lunch, instead of as a Square #5.

There's a lot of flexibility in the plan, which means even more choices for each meal!

After you have calculated the number of calories right for you to reach your health and weight-loss goals, you may make some combinations of meals accordingly. Some of the soups in Squares 2 and 4 have both a protein and a starch in them. If this is the case you may want to eliminate a starch from breakfast, dinner, or lunch.

Quick tip: I find it helps one feel more satisfied to add a tossed salad at dinnertime with your meal. Just don't forget the sugar-free dressing! Regular dressings often have a high sugar content.

Example of a simplified 5 square meal day:

BREAKFAST = eggs + potatoes + vegetables

MID-MORNING MEAL = tuna + salad

LUNCH = chicken + corn + vegetables

MIDDAY SNACK = turkey + vegetables

DINNER = fish + rice + vegetables, add dinner salad if desired

WHEN TO EAT

We have designed a typical day on 5 squares to equal no more than 1500 calories, which represents the approximate amount needed for a 150-pound female to lose a pound per week. Although five meals a day may seem like a lot, you actually burn more calories through digestion while eating so frequently.

Square #1

Breakfast: should be eaten within 20 minutes of rising. Breakfast is your metabolism's wake-up call each day (that's why it is literally the time to break the fast!). Some people can go until 2 or 3 P.M. before eating because their metabolism is still asleep. This is not healthy; in order for your body to burn calories efficiently, you want to get your metabolism working first thing in the morning. You will find after a few days that you feel a tremendous amount of energy at times when you used to feel sluggish.

Square #2

Mid-morning snack: should be eaten between 1½ and 3 hours after breakfast.

Square #3

Lunch: should be eaten 1½ to 3 hours after your mid-morning snack.

Square #4

Midday snack: should be eaten 1½ to 3 hours after your lunch.

Square #5

Dinner: should be eaten 1½ to 3 hours after your midday snack.

Helpful Tips:

- Here's a sample schedule based on the above guidelines:

  SQUARE #1: 7:30 A.M.

  SQUARE #2: 10:30 A.M.

  SQUARE #3: 1:30 P.M.

  SQUARE #4: 4:30 P.M.

  SQUARE #5: 7:30 P.M.

- A lot of people on the 5 squares plan tell me that they do not feel hungry at dinnertime anymore. Do not skip this meal. If you cannot finish your whole serving, do not, but this is the last meal you will consume before going to bed, and your body will digest it as you sleep.
  More digestion = more efficiency = burning more calories = more weight loss.

- When preparing the meals, package the second portion of your meals for the following day.

- Drink at least eight glasses of water a day. As on any diet, but especially high-protein diets, it's very important to stay hydrated.

- Refrain from alcoholic beverages and steer clear of milk, juices, and sodas that contain sugar. Opt for a sugar-free sweetener in your coffee or tea.

- Take a daily multivitamin and a calcium-zinc-magnesium supplement.

- For more information on staying on track while you're on the plan—including desirable and undesirable condiments, sugar-free sweeteners, and what to choose when dining out, please refer to Staying on Track: While You're on the Plan, page 181.

- The most important tip I can give you—stay focused! The first few days of any change may be difficult. You may experience a headache or even some fatigue. This is just a normal reaction to eliminating sugar, also known as "sugar withdrawal." By day 3 . . . you will feel spectacular!

FOOD DIARY

Individuals who keep a food diary are 60 percent more successful with weight loss than those who do not. It is important to keep a daily log of what we ingest to make us aware of unhealthy eating patterns. Be honest with yourself, and weigh yourself only once a week, at or around the same time of day. Jot down activities and exercises, as well.

Here is a sample food diary. I have included enough diaries for the next month; alternatively, you can download and print out the 5 squares food diary from our website: www.my5squares.com.

Example:

START DATE	SQUARE #1	SQUARE #2	SQUARE #3	SQUARE #4	SQUARE #5
MONDAY LIST ACTIVITY	• Steak and Eggs with Fresh Tomato Salsa • 1 cup decaffeinated tea	• Zesty Grilled Marinated Chicken Salad • 1 diet soft drink	• Turkey marinara • Bottle of water	• Tuna salad over greens • Bottle of water	• Orange Roughy Marinara with Caponata • 1 diet soft drink
TUESDAY LIST ACTIVITY Walked briskly 1 hour	• Perfect Hard-boiled Eggs with Oats • 1 cup decaffeinated tea	• Lentil Turkey Salad with Green Beans • Bottle of water	• Blue-Corn-Crusted salmon and sautéed vegetables • 1 diet soft drink	• Three-bean Salad • Bottle of water	• Oatmeal and almond-crusted pork tenderloin with asparagus • 1 diet soft drink
WEDNESDAY LIST ACTIVITY	• Spinach and Canadian bacon frittata • 5 squares Sautéed Breakfast Potatoes	• Crabmeat salad • Bottle of water	• Turkey cutlets with rosemary gravy • 1 diet soft drink	• Chicken and Roasted Pepper Salad over mixed greens • Bottle of water	• Stuffed Sole with Asparagus and Mushrooms • 1 diet soft drink

START DATE	SQUARE #1	SQUARE #2	SQUARE#3	SQUARE #4	SQUARE #5
THURSDAY LIST ACTIVITY Swam laps ½ hour	• Wheat-free French Toast with turkey sausage	• Italian Wedding Soup • Bottle of water	• Chicken Piccata with Steamed Asparagus • 1 bottle of diet tea	• Chicken Salad Lettuce Wrap • Bottle of water	• Chilean Sea Bass with Mint and Lemon Zest with Roasted Zucchini • 1 diet soft drink
FRIDAY WEIGHT 160 (−2) ☺ LIST ACTIVITY	• Button mushroom omelet • 5 squares Sautéed Breakfast Potatoes	• 5 squares Classic Split-Pea Soup with Canadian bacon	• Out to lunch— ordered grilled tuna steak with broccoli rabe • 1 diet soft drink	• Leftover tuna steak from lunch with small garden salad • Bottle of water	• Sesame-Crusted Sea Scallops with Thyme Roasted Potatoes and Sugar Snap Peas.
SATURDAY LIST ACTIVITY	• Wheat-free Strawberry Pancakes and turkey sausage • 1 cup decaffeinated tea	• Steamed salmon over mixed greens • 1 Cup decaffeinated tea	• Stuffed eggplant with mashed sweet potatoes • 1 diet soft drink	• Double Mustard Chicken and Arugula Salad • 1 bottle of diet tea	• Filet Mignon with and Garlic Mashed Potatoes and Sautéed Summer Squash • 1 diet soft drink
SUNDAY LIST ACTIVITY Raked lawn 1 hour	• Artichoke and Black Pepper Frittata • 5 squares Sautéed Breakfast Potatoes	• Roasted Garlic, Zucchini, and Chicken Soup • Bottle of water	• Stuffed peppers and braised cabbage • 1 diet soft drink	• Pulled Turkey Salad • Bottle of water	• Sautéed Tilapia with Black Bean Summer Squash Salad • 1 diet soft drink

START DATE	SQUARE #1	SQUARE #2	SQUARE #3	SQUARE #4	SQUARE #5
MONDAY LIST ACTIVITY					
TUESDAY LIST ACTIVITY					
WEDNESDAY LIST ACTIVITY					
THURSDAY LIST ACTIVITY					
FRIDAY WEIGHT_____ LIST ACTIVITY					
SATURDAY LIST ACTIVITY					
SUNDAY LIST ACTIVITY					

5 SQUARE LOW-CARB MEALS

START DATE	SQUARE #1	SQUARE #2	SQUARE #3	SQUARE #4	SQUARE #5
MONDAY LIST ACTIVITY					
TUESDAY LIST ACTIVITY					
WEDNESDAY LIST ACTIVITY					
THURSDAY LIST ACTIVITY					
FRIDAY WEIGHT_____ LIST ACTIVITY					
SATURDAY LIST ACTIVITY					
SUNDAY LIST ACTIVITY					

START DATE	SQUARE #1	SQUARE #2	SQUARE #3	SQUARE #4	SQUARE #5
MONDAY LIST ACTIVITY					
TUESDAY LIST ACTIVITY					
WEDNESDAY LIST ACTIVITY					
THURSDAY LIST ACTIVITY					
FRIDAY WEIGHT_____ LIST ACTIVITY					
SATURDAY LIST ACTIVITY					
SUNDAY LIST ACTIVITY					

START DATE	SQUARE #1	SQUARE #2	SQUARE #3	SQUARE #4	SQUARE #5
MONDAY LIST ACTIVITY					
TUESDAY LIST ACTIVITY					
WEDNESDAY LIST ACTIVITY					
THURSDAY LIST ACTIVITY					
FRIDAY WEIGHT_____ LIST ACTIVITY					
SATURDAY LIST ACTIVITY					
SUNDAY LIST ACTIVITY					

SAMPLE DAYS

Following are twenty sample days on the 5 squares diet. All of these recipes can be found in their numbered section. You should pick food items that you like and that are easy for you to prepare. I have always found that cooking meals ahead of time works best for planning and executing this lifestyle change. Purchase disposable food containers or Tupperware and package all of your next day's meals to take with you to work or to play. Do not get caught unprepared, as you may find that when it is time to eat, your only options are poor choices or fast foods.

If you find that you don't have time to prepare all your meals for a certain day, or you're faced with the challenge of eating out or on the go, please see pages 181–82 for helpful tips on quick grabs, dining out, and maintaining the good work you've done on the plan!

Day #1

SQUARE #1	Vermont Omelet
SQUARE #2	Perfect Shrimp Cocktail
SQUARE #3	Pesto-Grilled Chicken with Sautéed Cauliflower
SQUARE #4	Escarole and White Bean Soup
SQUARE #5	Stuffed Sole with Asparagus and Mushrooms served with Sautéed Sliced Potato and Onion

Day #2

SQUARE #1	Wheat-Free Blueberry Waffles (serve with turkey bacon and sugar-free maple syrup)
SQUARE #2	Barbecue Grilled Chicken with Sweet and Sour Cucumbers
SQUARE #3	Stuffed Eggplant with Mashed Sweet Potatoes
SQUARE #4	Chicken, Barley, and Vegetable Soup
SQUARE #5	Oatmeal-Almond-Crusted Flounder with Spicy Sautéed String Beans and Lemon Zest

Day #3

SQUARE #1	Mexican Scramble with Corn Tortillas
SQUARE #2	Pasta Fagiole

SQUARE #3	Beef Stir-Fry
SQUARE #4	Turkey Burger with Sautéed Mushrooms
SQUARE #5	Orange Roughy Marinara with Caponata

Day #4

SQUARE #1	Perfect Hard-Boiled Eggs with Cinnamon-Zested Oats
SQUARE #2	Turkey Salad with Chopped Apple, Tomato, and Romaine
SQUARE #3	Chicken Piccata with Steamed Asparagus and Savory Mushroom Brown Rice
SQUARE #4	Bean Salad with Canadian Bacon and Roasted Peppers
SQUARE #5	Chilean Sea Bass with Mint and Lemon Zest with Roasted Zucchini, Shallots, and Asparagus

Day #5

SQUARE #1	Steak and Eggs with Fresh Tomato Salsa
SQUARE #2	Spicy Lime and Cumin Marinated Chicken with Spinach
SQUARE #3	Grilled Marinated Lamb and Vegetables with Mint Pesto and Seasoned Barley
SQUARE #4	Three-Bean Salad
SQUARE #5	Orange Roughy Provençal with Rosemary-Roasted Potatoes

Day #6

SQUARE #1	Canadian Bacon and Spinach Soufflé
SQUARE #2	Fresh Crabmeat Salad
SQUARE #3	Turkey Cutlets with Rosemary Gravy, Garlic Mashed Potatoes, and Sautéed Sugar Snap Peas
SQUARE #4	Chicken and Roasted Pepper Salad
SQUARE #5	Sole à la Française with Sautéed Spinach

Day #7

    SQUARE #1   Artichoke and Black Pepper Frittata

    SQUARE #2   Roasted Garlic, Zucchini, and Chicken Soup

    SQUARE #3   Sautéed Tilapia with Black Bean and Corn Salad and Sautéed Broccoli Rabe

    SQUARE #4   Pulled Turkey Salad with Arugula, Garbanzos, and Red Onion

    SQUARE #5   Stuffed Chicken with Portobello and Spinach, Sweet Peas and Carrots

Day #8

    SQUARE #1   Wheat-Free Strawberry Pancakes (served with turkey sausage)

    SQUARE #2   Steamed Salmon Fillet over Mesclun Greens

    SQUARE #3   Shrimp à la Française with Sweet Peas and Carrots

    SQUARE #4   Double-Mustard Chicken and Arugula Salad

    SQUARE #5   Filet Mignon with Garlic Mashed Potatoes and Sautéed Summer Squash

Day #9

    SQUARE #1   Spanish Scramble

    SQUARE #2   Waldorf Chicken Salad with Raspberry Vinaigrette

    SQUARE #3   Stuffed Flank Steak with Spinach and Onions over Seasoned Barley

    SQUARE #4   Turkey Burger with Grilled Eggplant and Sautéed Zucchini

    SQUARE #5   Grilled Mahimahi with Julienned Vegetables and Pineapple Salsa

Day #10

    SQUARE #1   Wheat-Free Banana Nut Waffles (served with turkey sausage links)

    SQUARE #2   Shrimp and White Bean Salad

SQUARE #3	Marinated Fajita with Sautéed Broccoli and Baked Sliced Sweet Potato
SQUARE #4	Chicken Sautéed with Peppers, Eggplant, and Mushrooms
SQUARE #5	Veal and Pepper Stew à la Marinara with Brown Rice

Day #11

SQUARE #1	Canadian Bacon, Mushroom, and Onion Scramble
SQUARE #2	Chicken Salad with Cucumbers, Tomatoes, and Basil
SQUARE #3	Turkey Meatloaf with Sautéed Spinach and Mashed Potatoes
SQUARE #4	Barbequed Salmon with Braised Cabbage
SQUARE #5	Chicken Quesadilla with Fresh Tomato Salsa and White Bean and Artichoke Dip

Day #12

SQUARE #1	Zucchini and Black Pepper Scramble
SQUARE #2	Balsamic Marinated Chicken Strips with Mixed Greens
SQUARE #3	Stuffed Peppers with Herbed Tomato Sauce and Braised Cabbage
SQUARE #4	Seafood Salad
SQUARE #5	Horseradish-and-Oat-Crusted Pork Loin with Rosemary Gravy

Day #13

SQUARE #1	Button Mushroom Omelet
SQUARE #2	5 Squares Classic Split-Pea Soup
SQUARE #3	Turkey Marinara over Brown Rice
SQUARE #4	Chicken Salad Lettuce Wrap
SQUARE #5	Sesame-Crusted Sea Scallops with Thyme-Roasted Potatoes and Sautéed Sugar Snap Peas

Day #14

SQUARE #1   Wheat-Free French Toast with Strawberries and Canadian Bacon

SQUARE #2   Italian Wedding Soup with Turkey Meatballs and Escarole

SQUARE #3   Lemon-Garlic Chicken with Rosemary-Roasted Potatoes and Sautéed String Beans Almandine

SQUARE #4   Pesto Shrimp Cocktail

SQUARE #5   Turkey Vegetable Stir-Fry with Rice Noodles

Day #15

SQUARE #1   Shrimp, Scallion, and Asparagus Omelets

SQUARE #2   Mushroom, Beef, and Barley Soup

SQUARE #3   Spicy Catfish with Roasted Fennel and Sautéed Green Beans

SQUARE #4   Julienned Turkey Chef Salad

SQUARE #5   Chicken Rollatini with Savory Mushroom Brown Rice

Day #16

SQUARE #1   Wheat-Free Banana Nut Muffins (served with turkey bacon)

SQUARE #2   Fresh Salmon Salad with Capers and Dill

SQUARE #3   Turkey Meatballs à la Marinara with Brown Rice Ziti

SQUARE #4   Pulled Chicken Salad with Peppers, Eggplant, and Spelt Croutons

SQUARE #5   Garlic-and-Herb Crusted Pork with Roasted Butternut Squash and Sautéed Broccoli Rabe

Day #17

SQUARE #1   Smoky Turkey and Spinach Omelets

SQUARE #2   Lentil Turkey Salad with Green Beans

SQUARE #3   Baked Spice-Rubbed Salmon with Sautéed Spinach

SQUARE #4   Spicy Roasted Pepper Soup with Chicken and Lime

SQUARE #5   Chicken Rollatini with Roasted Peppers and Asparagus

Day #18

SQUARE #1	Sausage, Pepper, and Onion Scramble
SQUARE #2	5 Squares Tuna Salad
SQUARE #3	Mustard-Baked Swordfish with Quick Tomato Salsa and Steamed Broccoli
SQUARE #4	Chicken, Cauliflower, and Leek Soup
SQUARE #5	Baked Chicken with Sautéed Escarole and Spicy Asian Rice Noodles

Day #19

SQUARE #1	Baked Apples and Canadian Bacon
SQUARE #2	Zesty Grilled Marinated Chicken Salad
SQUARE #3	Roast Pork Loin with Fresh Herbs and Roasted Vegetables
SQUARE #4	Balsamic-Glazed Tuna with Spicy Cucumber Salad
SQUARE #5	Turkey Chili with Sautéed Potatoes

Day #20

SQUARE #1	Potato and Chive Frittata
SQUARE #2	Fresh Whitefish Salad with Cucumbers and Red Onion Vinaigrette
SQUARE #3	Blue-Corn-Crusted Salmon with Spicy, Sautéed Vegetable Medley
SQUARE #4	Chopped Chicken Salad with Creamy Lemon-Dill Vinaigrette
SQUARE #5	Stuffed Tomatoes with Garlic Sautéed Broccoli

LYNN MITCHELL'S 5 SQUARES
MAKEOVER SUCCESS STORY

I PUT MYSELF ON MY FIRST diet when I was 15 and my parents had forced me to go to modeling school in suburban Philadelphia. I was five four and although I wasn't unattractive, I wore a solid size 8 and was not necessarily runway material like some of the other girls. I hated being "the big girl" and felt very self-conscious.

I began to eat less and joined a cross-country team. My coach realized something was wrong when I fainted one day during practice. I confessed to him that I hadn't really been eating, and after a bit of intervention by him and my family, I was back on three meals a day. Even with the running, I found my weight slowly creeping up and by the time I entered college, I was wearing a size ten.

At college, I started using food as an emotional barometer. If I was happy, I ate. If I was upset, I ate. If I was nervous, I ate. I especially loved ice cream and chocolate chip cookies: the bad stuff. By the end of my first year, I had put an additional "freshman 20" on top of my already challenged frame. I spent that summer at home and with the help of my parents and a sensible exercise regime, I lost the excess weight.

The next year was a tragic one for me, however. At school I fell victim to date rape. Although I went to therapy, I never truly got over the feeling that somehow, my body was responsible for what had happened to me. I kept myself a good 10 to 20 pounds overweight as a safety net, so if a guy was interested in me, I'd know it wasn't for my looks or my body.

Around that time I began a downward spiral of binge eating. I would go to the local market or even the school commissary and return to my dorm with bags of food, then consume them all in a 30-minute sprint. This self-destructive behavior continued even after I graduated and moved to New York.

Despite my self-abusive behavior, I still managed to maintain a size 10. But when I turned 35, everything changed. It appeared as though everything I ate, healthy or unhealthy, would remain on my hips, thighs, and butt. I tried to ignore the fact that every three months or so, I would go up another dress size. By the time I approached my thirty-sixth birthday, I had become a size eighteen.

I put myself on a restricted diet and exercised like a mad woman. Four weeks later, I had lost only 3 pounds. I started freaking out. Why wasn't I losing the weight? My mother blamed it on my age. Like all daughters, I refused to believe her. I doubled my efforts, cutting even more calories, and spending more time exercising. The result? Four weeks later, I had only lost another 3 pounds and had developed shin splints. I was so depressed that I stayed in on my thirty-sixth birthday: instead of kicking up my heels I stayed home crying and feeling sorry for myself. That night was a turning point in my life. I ended up on the computer and through a Web search found Monica Lynn and 5 squares.

I began that very next day. I was surprised that the food was so delicious and abundant. I especially loved the Horseradish-and-Oat-Crusted Pork Loin [see page 159] (what can I say, I'm part German!).

My friends and family could not believe that I was eating so healthily and actually enjoying it. They had seen me on countless diets over the years, and I hadn't exactly been the most cheerful dieter. I explained to them that this was not a diet, but a lifestyle change. I was doing something positive instead of beating my body into submission.

I have to admit the first week was a challenge. I really had to retrain my mind and my body. I had been a "sugar addict" (M&Ms were my best friends for years) and it took a few days to get the sugar out of my body. Once this happened though, I found that I didn't want it or crave it anymore. My moods were steadier and I no longer had trouble staying alert during the day or sleeping at night. My skin even cleared up and in two weeks, I had lost 12 pounds. I was so thrilled I treated myself to a new dress and a spa massage. I liked rewarding myself with something other than food for once.

As happy as I was with the weight loss, I was also pleased that I was finally on my way to a healthy new life and a new way of eating.

In six and a half months, I lost the 60 pounds that had once felt like a barrier between me and the world. I revamped my wardrobe, met a guy, and found a new mindset. I am now the proud new owner of a great body, and an even greater attitude.

RECIPES

NOTE: Many of the recipes in this book are designed to serve two people. If you are starting this program by yourself, I recommend saving the second portion for the next day.

Also, I have provided nutritional information for each square. This includes all sides that are served with the recipe.

Happy Eating!

SQUARE 1

Zucchini and Black Pepper Scramble

SERVES 2

SERVE WITH 5 SQUARES SAUTÉED BREAKFAST POTATOES (PAGE 37)

1 teaspoon olive oil

1 cup thinly sliced zucchini, about 4 ounces

½ teaspoon salt

¼ teaspoon coarse ground black pepper

12 ounces egg whites, about 1½ cups

1   Heat a medium nonstick skillet over medium-high heat until hot. Add the oil, zucchini, salt, and pepper, and stir-fry for 2 to 3 minutes until lightly browned.

2   Add the egg whites to the pan and scramble until cooked through, about 2 minutes.

PER SERVING, WITH POTATOES:

176 calories	24 g protein	14 g total carbohydrates	2 g fiber	12 g net carbohydrates

5 SQUARES SAUTÉED BREAKFAST POTATOES

SERVES 2

1 teaspoon olive oil

1 small Idaho potato, about 8 ounces, uncooked, peeled, and
sliced into ½-inch cubes

½ cup low-sodium chicken stock

Salt and fresh ground black pepper to taste

1   Heat a medium nonstick skillet over medium heat until hot. Add the oil and
    potato. Raise the heat to medium-high and sauté 3 to 5 minutes, stirring fre-
    quently until the potatoes are well browned.

2   Add the chicken stock and reduce the heat to low. Cover the skillet and sim-
    mer until the stock has been absorbed and the potatoes are tender, about 6 to
    8 minutes. Season with salt and pepper and serve.

Steak and Eggs with Fresh Tomato Salsa

SERVE WITH 5 SQUARES SAUTÉED BREAKFAST POTATOES
(PAGE 37)

 1 teaspoon olive oil

 4 ounces store-bought packaged beef strips for stir-fry

 ¼ teaspoon salt

 ⅛ teaspoon fresh ground black pepper

 12 ounces egg whites, about 1½ cups

1 Preheat the oven to 200° F.

2 Heat a medium nonstick skillet over medium-high heat until hot. Add the oil, beef, salt, and pepper and stir-fry for 2 to 3 minutes until cooked through. Remove the skillet from the heat. Transfer the steak to plates and keep warm in the oven.

3 Wipe the skillet out, then lightly coat it with nonstick cooking spray (preferably Pam). Return the skillet to the heat, add the egg whites to the pan, and scramble until set, 1 to 2 minutes. Serve the eggs and steak topped with the salsa (page 39).

PER SERVING, WITH POTATOES:

240 calories	31 g protein	13 g total carbohydrates	1 g fiber	12 g net carbohydrates

FRESH TOMATO SALSA

2 plum tomatoes, diced, about ⅔ cup

¼ teaspoon dried oregano

1 clove garlic, crushed to a paste

1 tablespoon chopped fresh cilantro

1 tablespoon lemon juice

Tabasco or hot sauce to taste

Pinch of salt

In a bowl combine the tomatoes, oregano, garlic, cilantro, and lemon juice. Season with a few drops of the Tabasco and the salt.

Potato and Chive Frittata

1 small russet or Yukon Gold potato, about 8 ounces

1 tablespoon fresh lemon juice

1 teaspoon olive oil

Salt and fresh ground black pepper to taste

12 ounces egg whites, about 1½ cups

2 tablespoons finely cut chives

1. Preheat the oven to 375°F. Lightly coat an 8-inch ovenproof nonstick skillet with nonstick cooking spray (preferably Pam).

2. Peel and slice the potatoes into thin bite-size pieces. Place in a separate medium-size saucepan with water to cover. Cover pan and steam the potatoes for 7 to 8 minutes until tender.

3. Toss the potatoes with the lemon juice and olive oil. Season with the salt and pepper and spread in the prepared skillet.

4. Place the egg whites in a bowl and whisk in the chives. Season with salt and pepper.

5. Pour the egg whites into the pan.

6. Transfer the pan to the middle shelf of the oven for 20 minutes until the eggs are set.

7. Run a thin flexible spatula around the edge of the frittata to loosen it. Place a plate over the skillet and invert the frittata.

8. Slice into wedges and serve.

PER SERVING:

124 calories	23 g protein	13.8 g total carbohydrates	1 g fiber	12.8 g net carbohydrates

Spanish Scramble

SERVE WITH 5 SQUARES SAUTÉED BREAKFAST POTATOES
(PAGE 37).

12 ounces egg whites, about 1½ cups

1 tablespoon shredded soy cheese

Salt and pepper to taste

1 small onion, thinly sliced, about ½ cup

½ medium yellow bell pepper, cored and chopped, about ½ cup

1 medium tomato, cored and chopped, about ½ cup

1   Place the egg whites in a bowl. Whisk in the soy cheese. Season with salt and pepper.

2   Lightly coat a medium nonstick skillet with Pam and place over medium heat.

3   Add the onion and sauté 2 to 3 minutes, stirring occasionally until lightly browned.

4   Add the pepper and tomato and sauté 2 to 3 minutes until soft.

5   Stir in the egg white mixture and scramble until cooked through, about 2 minutes. Serve hot.

PER SERVING, WITH POTATOES:

188 calories	27.5 g protein	19 g total carbohydrates	4 g fiber	15 g net carbohydrates

Mexican Scramble
with Corn Tortillas

Two 6-inch fresh corn tortillas

12 ounces egg whites, about 1½ cups

Salt and fresh ground black pepper to taste

1 recipe Fresh Tomato Salsa (page 39)

2 tablespoons grated soy cheese (optional)

1   Heat a griddle over medium heat until hot. Toast the tortillas 1 to 2 minutes per side until crisp.

2   Heat a medium nonstick skillet over medium heat until hot. Add the egg whites and scramble until cooked through. Season with salt and pepper.

3   Place the tortillas on plates, top with the eggs, salsa, and a sprinkle of cheese if desired. Serve immediately.

PER SERVING:

164 calories	24 g protein	14 g total carbohydrates	2 g fiber	12 g net carbohydrates

Canadian Bacon, Mushroom, and Onion Scramble

SERVES 2

SERVE WITH 5 SQUARES SAUTÉED POTATOES (PAGE 37).

12 ounces egg whites, about 1½ cups

2 teaspoons finely chopped fresh parsley

3 ounces Canadian bacon, diced, about ¾ cup

1 small onion, thinly sliced, about ½ cup

4 ounces mushrooms, thinly sliced, about 2 cups

Salt and fresh ground black pepper to taste

1   Whisk the egg whites and parsley in a small bowl to combine.

2   Lightly coat a medium nonstick skillet with Pam and place over medium heat.

3   Add the bacon, onion, and mushrooms and sauté 3 to 4 minutes, stirring occasionally until lightly browned.

4   Stir in the egg white mixture and scramble until cooked through, about 2 minutes. Season with salt and pepper and serve.

PER SERVING, WITH POTATOES:

239 calories	35 g protein	17.5 g total carbohydrates	3 g fiber	14.5 g net carbohydrates

Sausage, Pepper, and Onion Scramble

SERVES 2

SERVE WITH 5 SQUARES SAUTÉED BREAKFAST POTATOES
(PAGE 37)

12 ounces egg whites, about 1½ cups

1 teaspoon chopped fresh sage

Four 1-ounce turkey sausage links, sliced into ½-inch pieces

1 small onion, thinly sliced, about ½ cup

1 medium red bell pepper, diced, about 1 cup

Salt and fresh ground black pepper to taste

1   Whisk the egg whites and sage in a small bowl to combine.

2   Lightly coat a medium nonstick skillet with Pam and place over medium heat.

3   Add the sausage, onion, and pepper and sauté 3 to 4 minutes, stirring occasionally until lightly browned.

4   Stir in the egg white mixture and scramble until cooked through, about 2 minutes. Season with salt and pepper and serve.

PER SERVING, WITH POTATOES:

203 calories	34 g protein	19 g total carbohydrates	3 g fiber	16 g net carbohydrates

Button Mushroom Omelets

SERVE WITH 5 SQUARES SAUTÉED BREAKFAST POTATOES
(PAGE 37)

12 ounces egg whites, about 1½ cups

Salt and fresh ground black pepper to taste

4 ounces button mushrooms, thinly sliced, about 2 cups

1   Place the egg whites in a bowl. Season with salt and pepper.

2   Lightly coat a medium nonstick skillet with Pam and place over medium heat.

3   Add the mushrooms and sauté 3 to 5 minutes, stirring occasionally until lightly browned. Remove the skillet from the heat, season the mushrooms with salt and pepper, and set aside in a bowl.

4   Wipe out the skillet, and lightly coat it with Pam. Return the skillet to the heat and pour in half of the egg whites, reserving the other half for the second omelet. Cook until barely set. Spoon half of the mushrooms over one half of the egg whites in the pan. With a spatula loosen the other half of the egg whites and fold it over the mushrooms. Cook for a minute, then flip and continue to cook until cooked through.

5   Make a second omelet with the remaining ingredients.

PER SERVING, WITH POTATOES:

171 calories	25 g protein	13.8 g total carbohydrates	1.5 g fiber	12.3 g net carbohydrates

Vermont Omelets

SERVE WITH 5 SQUARES SAUTÉED BREAKFAST POTATOES
(PAGE 37)

3 ounces Canadian bacon, diced, about ¾ cup

½ cup chopped red or green apple

2 cups prewashed baby spinach

Salt and fresh ground black pepper to taste

12 ounces egg whites, about 1½ cups

2 tablespoons shredded soy cheddar

1   Lightly coat a medium nonstick skillet with Pam and place over medium heat.

2   Add the bacon and apple. Sauté 2 to 3 minutes, stirring occasionally until lightly browned. Add the spinach and stir until wilted, about 1 minute. Remove the skillet from the heat, season the mixture with salt and pepper, and place it in a bowl.

3   Wipe out the skillet, and lightly coat it with Pam. Return the pan to the heat, pour in half of the egg whites, and immediately sprinkle entirely with half of the soy cheddar. Cook until barely set.

4   Spoon half of the apple-bacon-spinach filling over one half of the egg whites in the skillet. Loosen the other half of the egg white with a spatula and fold it over the filling. Cook for a minute, then flip and cook through.

5   Make a second omelet with the remaining ingredients.

PER SERVING, WITH POTATOES:

250 calories	31 g protein	17 g total carbohydrates	3 g fiber	14 g net carbohydrates

Shrimp, Scallion, and Asparagus Omelets

SERVES 2

SERVE WITH 5 SQUARES SAUTÉED BREAKFAST POTATOES
(PAGE 37)

12 ounces egg whites, about 1½ cups

3 to 4 scallions, thinly sliced, about ½ cup

Salt and fresh ground black pepper to taste

4 ounces shrimp, peeled, deveined, and sliced into ½-inch pieces

8 slender asparagus spears, trimmed and sliced into 1-inch lengths

1 Place the egg whites and scallions in a bowl. Season with the salt and pepper and whisk to combine.

2 Lightly coat a medium nonstick skillet with Pam and place over medium heat.

3 Add the shrimp and asparagus and sauté 3 to 5 minutes until the shrimp are cooked through and the asparagus are slightly tender. Remove the skillet from the heat, season with salt and pepper, and set the mixture aside in a bowl.

4 Wipe out the skillet and lightly coat it with Pam. Return the pan to the heat and pour in half of the egg whites. Cook until barely set. Spoon half of the shrimp and asparagus over one half of the egg whites in the skillet. With a spatula, loosen the other half of the egg whites and fold it over the vegetables. Cook for a minute, then flip and continue to cook until cooked through.

5 Make a second omelet with the remaining ingredients.

PER SERVING, WITH POTATOES:

235 calories	36 g protein	16 g total carbohydrates	3 g fiber	13 g net carbohydrates

Smoky Turkey and Spinach Omelets

SERVES 2

SERVE WITH 5 SQUARES SAUTÉED BREAKFAST POTATOES (PAGE 37)

> 4 strips uncooked turkey bacon, sliced into ½-inch strips
>
> 2 ounces fresh prewashed spinach
>
> 12 ounces egg whites, about 1½ cups

1   Preheat the oven to 375°F.

2   Lightly spray a medium nonstick skillet with Pam. Place over medium heat.

3   When the skillet is hot, add the bacon and sauté 2 to 3 minutes until lightly browned. Add the spinach and sauté until wilted, about 1 minute. Remove the skillet from the heat and transfer the mixture to a plate.

4   Wipe out the skillet and lightly coat it with Pam. Return it to the heat and pour in half of the egg whites. Cook until barely set. Spoon half of the bacon and spinach over one half of the egg whites in the skillet. Loosen the other half of the egg whites with a spatula and fold it over the vegetables. Cook for a minute, then flip and continue to cook until cooked through.

5   Make a second omelet with the remaining ingredients.

PER SERVING, WITH POTATOES:

205 calories	30 g protein	13 g total carbohydrates	2 g fiber	11 g net carbohydrates

Canadian Bacon and Spinach Frittata

SERVE WITH 5 SQUARES SAUTÉED BREAKFAST POTATOES
(PAGE 37)

> 3 ounces diced Canadian bacon, about ¾ cup
>
> 2 ounces prewashed baby spinach
>
> 12 ounces egg whites, about 1½ cups
>
> Salt and fresh ground black pepper to taste

1   Preheat the oven to 375°F.

2   Heat an 8-inch ovenproof, nonstick skillet over medium heat until hot. Add the bacon and sauté 3 to 5 minutes, stirring occasionally until lightly browned. Add the spinach and cook 1 to 2 minutes until wilted.

3   While the spinach cooks, place the egg whites, salt, and pepper in a mixing bowl and beat until they hold soft peaks. Spread the egg whites over the bacon and spinach in the skillet.

4   Transfer the frittata to the middle shelf of the oven and bake for 20 minutes until golden brown and cooked through.

PER SERVING, WITH POTATOES:

219 calories	34 g protein	16 g total carbohydrates	3 g fiber	13 g net carbohydrates

Artichoke and Black Pepper Frittata

SERVES 2

SERVE WITH 5 SQUARES SAUTÉED BREAKFAST POTATOES
(PAGE 37)

4 to 5 canned artichoke hearts, drained and thinly sliced

12 ounces egg whites, about 1½ cups

½ teaspoon salt

¼ teaspoon fresh ground black pepper

1 Preheat the oven to 375°F. Lightly coat an 8-inch ovenproof nonstick skillet with Pam.

2 Spread the artichokes over the skillet.

3 In a small bowl combine the egg whites, salt, and pepper and whisk until soft peaks form.

4 Pour the egg whites into the skillet and place it on middle shelf of the oven.

5 Bake for 20 minutes until set.

6 Run a thin, flexible spatula around the edge of the frittata to loosen it. Place a plate over the skillet and invert the frittata.

7 Slice into wedges and serve.

PER SERVING, WITH POTATOES:

168 calories	24 g protein	15 g total carbohydrates	2 g fiber	13 g net carbohydrates

Perfect Hard-Boiled Eggs
with Cinnamon-Zested Oats

4 large eggs

1   Gently place the eggs in a small saucepan. Cover the eggs with cold water and place the pan over high heat.

2   When the water reaches a boil, cover the pan and turn off the heat.

3   After 12 minutes, drain the eggs. Gently crack each of the eggs all over against the side of the sink and place them in a bowl of cold water to cool for approximately 10 minutes. Peel and serve with Cinnamon-Zested Oats (below).

CINNAMON-ZESTED OATS

2 cups water

1 cup quick-cooking rolled oats (1 minute, not instant)

Pinch of ground cinnamon

2 packages Splenda (sugar-free sweetener), if desired

Bring the 2 cups water to a boil in a small saucepan. Add the oats and cinnamon. Reduce the heat and simmer for 2 to 3 minutes, stirring occasionally until the oats have thickened to a creamy mass. If you like sweeter oatmeal, 2 packages of Splenda work beautifully. Serve with the hard-boiled eggs or if you prefer, turkey sausage (4 links per serving).

PER SERVING:

290 calories	17 g protein	29 g total carbohydrates	4 g fiber	25 g net carbohydrates

Baked Apples and Canadian Bacon

2 medium red apples, halved and cored

½ cup water

2 teaspoons lemon juice

2 packages Splenda (sugar-free sweetener)

¼ cup Maple Grove Farms Cozy Cottage Sugar Free Syrup

½ teaspoons ground cinnamon

4 ounces Canadian bacon, thinly sliced

1 Preheat the oven to 375°F.

2 Place the apples cut side up in a baking dish large enough to hold them in a single snug layer.

3 Pour the water around the apples.

4 Sprinkle the apples with lemon juice and Splenda. Drizzle with syrup and dust with ground cinnamon.

5 Bake 20 to 30 minutes until tender but not falling apart.

6 Heat a medium nonstick grill pan or skillet over medium heat until hot. Fry the bacon about 1 minute on each side, until heated through. Serve with the warm apples.

PER SERVING:

166 calories	12 g protein	20 g total carbohydrates	3 g fiber	17 g net carbohydrates

Wheat-Free
Banana-Nut Waffles

SERVE WITH TURKEY SAUSAGES OR TURKEY BACON
(4 LINKS OR 4 STRIPS PER SERVING)

½ cup Arrowhead Mills Wheat Free All Purpose Baking Mix

⅓ cup coarsely chopped walnuts

⅓ cup unsweetened soy milk (we use VITASOY brand)

1 large egg

1 teaspoon vanilla extract

½ package Splenda (sugar-free sweetener)

½ banana, sliced into thin rounds

Sugar-free syrup to taste (we use Maple Grove Farms Cozy Cottage brand)

1   Lightly spray a standard four-section waffle iron with Pam and heat it.

2   Combine the wheat-free baking mix and chopped walnuts in a bowl.

3   In a second bowl, whisk the soy milk, egg, vanilla, and Splenda until smooth. Pour the liquids into the dry mix and stir to form a smooth batter.

4   Pour enough batter just to fill the waffle iron and top with 3 to 4 slices of banana. Bake the waffles until lightly brown, approximately 5 minutes.

5   Repeat with the remaining batter. Serve warm.

PER SERVING, WITH MEAT:

200 calories	10 g protein	21 g total carbohydrates	2 g fiber	18.65 g net carbohydrates

Wheat-Free
Blueberry Waffles

SERVES 4 (TWO WAFFLE SECTIONS PER PERSON)

SERVE WITH TURKEY SAUSAGES OR TURKEY BACON
(4 LINKS OR 4 STRIPS PER SERVING)

⅓ cup unsweetened soy milk (we use VITASOY brand)

1 large egg

1 teaspoon vanilla extract

1 teaspoon finely grated orange or lemon zest (optional)

½ package Splenda (sugar-free sweetener)

½ cup Arrowhead Mills Wheat Free All Purpose Baking Mix

½ cup blueberries (fresh or frozen)

Sugar-free syrup to taste (such as Maple Grove Farms Cozy Cottage)

1   Lightly spray a standard four-section waffle iron with Pam and heat it.

2   In a bowl whisk the soy milk, egg, vanilla extract, zest, and Splenda until smooth. Add the baking mix and stir to form a smooth batter.

3   Pour enough batter just to fill waffle iron and top with 6 to 8 blueberries. Bake the waffles until lightly brown, approximately 5 minutes.

4   Repeat with the remaining batter. Serve warm.

PER SERVING, WITH MEAT:

161 calories	14 g protein	18 g total carbohydrates	1 g fiber	17 g net carbohydrates

Wheat-Free French Toast with Strawberries and Canadian Bacon

4 egg whites, about 1 cup

½ cup unflavored soy milk (we use VITASOY brand)

¼ cup water

1 teaspoon vanilla extract

¼ teaspoon ground cinnamon

½ teaspoon Splenda (sugar-free sweetener)

4 slices whole meal spelt bread (we use Baldwin Hill brand)

Sugar-free syrup to taste (such as Maple Grove Farms Cozy Cottage)

3 to 4 sliced strawberries for garnish

4 ounces Canadian bacon, thinly sliced (you can substitute turkey sausages or bacon, 4 links or 4 strips per serving)

1   In a mixing bowl whisk together the egg whites, soy milk, water, vanilla, cinnamon, and Splenda.

2   Lay the bread in a baking dish large enough to hold the slices in a single snug layer.

3   Pour the egg white mixture over the bread and turn to coat. Set aside for 15 to 20 minutes to allow the bread to soften and soak up the flavorings.

4   Lightly spray a large nonstick skillet with Pam and place over medium heat.

5   Transfer the bread to the pan and cook 2 to 3 minutes per side until golden brown. Drizzle with the sugar-free syrup and garnish with the sliced strawberries.

6   Heat a medium nonstick grill pan or skillet over medium heat until hot. Fry the Canadian bacon until heated through, about 1 minute on each side. Serve next to the French toast.

PER SERVING:

267 calories	33 g protein	46 g total carbohydrates	5 g fiber	41 g net carbohydrates

Wheat-Free Banana-Nut Muffins

MAKES 8 TO 9 MUFFINS. RECOMMENDED SERVING SIZE IS 1 MUFFIN PER PERSON.

SERVE WITH 4 OUNCES OF CANADIAN BACON, 8 STRIPS OF
TURKEY BACON (4 STRIPS PER SERVING), OR 8 LINKS OF
TURKEY SAUSAGES (4 LINKS PER SERVING). LEFTOVER
MUFFINS FREEZE BEAUTIFULLY FOR UP TO 1 MONTH.

1¾ cups Arrowhead Mills All Purpose Wheat Free Baking Mix

½ teaspoon baking powder

½ cup chopped walnuts

1 egg, lightly beaten

¼ cup unsweetened soy milk (we use VITASOY brand)

¼ cup canola oil

6 tablespoons Maple Grove Farms Cozy Cottage Sugar Free Maple Syrup

1 ripe banana, mashed

1 teaspoon vanilla extract

2 teaspoons finely grated orange zest

1 Preheat the oven to 350°F.

2 In a medium bowl combine the wheat-free baking mix, baking powder, and walnuts.

3 In a blender combine the egg, soy milk, oil, syrup, banana, vanilla, and orange zest. Puree until smooth.

4 Pour the puree into the dry baking mix and stir to combine.

5 Lightly spray a nonstick standard-size muffin pan with Pam. Drop ⅓ cup batter into each muffin compartment.

6 Bake for 20 to 25 minutes until a toothpick inserted in the center of a muffin comes out clean.

PER SERVING, WITH MEAT:

315 calories	14 g protein	21 g total carbohydrates	2 g fiber	19 g net carbohydrates

Wheat-Free Strawberry Pancakes

SERVE WITH TURKEY SAUSAGES OR TURKEY BACON
(4 LINKS OR STRIPS PER SERVING)

1 large egg

⅓ cup unsweetened soy milk (we use VITASOY brand)

1 teaspoon vanilla extract

⅛ teaspoon Splenda (sugar-free sweetener)

½ cup Arrowhead Mills Wheat Free All Purpose Baking Mix

2 to 3 strawberries, hulled and thinly sliced

1 In a bowl whisk the egg with the soy milk, vanilla, and Splenda. Add the baking mix and whisk until smooth.

2 Lightly spray a large nonstick griddle or skillet with Pam and place it over medium heat.

3 Pour ⅓ cup of the batter at a time to form four pancakes (you may have to do this two pancakes at a time if your skillet is small). Cook until bubbles appear and immediately add 3 to 4 slices of strawberries to each pancake. Cook for a few seconds more before flipping the pancakes. Cook until golden brown and serve with sugar-free syrup.

PER SERVING, WITH MEAT:

249 calories	18 g protein	30 g total carbohydrates	3 g fiber	27 g net carbohydrates

STACEY LEI'S 5 SQUARES
MAKEOVER SUCCESS STORY

I AM A FITNESS EDUCATOR IN New York City, and have been training people to
live active lifestyles for over 15 years. I have never claimed to be a nutritionist and
have outsourced dietary professionals for my clients when necessary. My focus is to
train fitness instructors to motivate their clients through movement, and to inspire my
own clients to integrate movement into their lives. My chiropractor, Dr. Patrick Eglauf,
has always said "Movement is Life" and I've adapted this as my own philosophy.
Without a question, I am physically active from the first hour of my day until I lie
down at night.

As a result of this intense lifestyle, I have been struggling with my weight for almost
10 years . . . but not in the traditional sense. I struggle to *keep weight on.* Of course,
the average person will have an issue with my true confession; however, the reality
is . . . a weight problem is a weight problem. At times, I've found myself actively
training for 6 to 8 hours each day. In between my aggressive gigs, transportation in
New York City means walking, stair climbing, and rollerblading. . . . so I'm basically
burning calories at an incredible rate. When I met with Monica Lynn about my
concerns, she had me do exactly what I've asked of my clients, journal my food intake
for 7 days.

I was amazed at what I found. Although I was eating tremendous amounts of food, I
was always filling up with carbohydrates. I was constantly craving hi-carb snacks
(mainly fruits) and eating big bowls of pasta for dinner, mixed with small portions of
veggies and protein. I felt justified eating what I craved; since I worked so hard, I
deserved to eat my comfort foods. I felt that the nighttime carb-loading would
provide me with the energy I required to carry me through the next day. Little did I
realize that I was simply stuck in a horrible sugar cycle . . . the more I ate, the more I
craved . . . and then I would just crash from exhaustion. The food was not sustaining
me. I was constantly tired, and never able to gain the weight that I needed to stay
strong and energized though my workouts.

I started on 5 squares soon after Monica told me about her program. The food was
amazing, but I found a few challenges. The meals seemed so small at first! (Then I
recognized that they were actually what *serving sizes* are supposed to be, instead of

¾ pound of pasta.) Getting off carbohydrates was tough for me too—it took me 3 full days until I didn't crave pasta or bread! Soon, however, my life began to change.

I followed the 5 squares plan every day for 2 weeks, and then Monica suggested that I double my protein intake to sustain my high levels of physical activity. This was my turning point. Over the next 3 weeks, I gained 5 pounds of lean muscle mass (the most in years) and I had an abundance of energy. I was fully functional and active on only 6 hours of sleep per night (instead of 8). I no longer needed afternoon naps or caffeine to get me though my toughest workouts. I was stronger than ever. My clients all noticed my increased energy, and they began the program . . . to help them lose weight. Everyone who stuck with the program was successful.

5 squares changed my life. I have now begun to cook my own meals, but I focus on clean food: low-carb solutions and appropriate portion sizes. I'm no longer tempted to order cream-based sauces and overly rich foods when I dine out. Although my entire philosophy of fitness and wellness is balance, I recognize that 5 squares helped me to truly understand and apply a balanced, healthy eating routine to my own life.

We all must remember this: what we put in, we get out . . . and all of our goals are within our reach—we just need to be brave enough to make a change.

Italian Wedding Soup
with Turkey Meatballs
and Escarole

FOR THE TURKEY MEATBALLS:

6 ounces ground turkey

2 tablespoons sugar-free marinara sauce

1 teaspoon egg white

1 tablespoon finely ground oatmeal or oat flour

1 teaspoon chopped parsley

2 teaspoons chopped basil

½ teaspoon dried oregano

¼ teaspoon salt

1 teaspoon olive oil

1 tablespoon minced onion

1 clove garlic, crushed

1   Preheat the oven to 375°F.

2   In a bowl combine the turkey, marinara sauce, egg white, oatmeal or flour, parsley, basil, oregano, and salt.

3   Warm the oil in a 6- to 8-inch nonstick skillet over medium heat. Add the onion and garlic and sauté 1 to 2 minutes until golden brown.

4   Transfer the onion mixture to the bowl with the turkey and mix well.

5   Form the mixture into six balls.

6   Lightly spray a baking sheet with Pam. Transfer the balls to the pan and bake for 20 minutes or until cooked through. Turn the balls halfway through for even browning.

1 teaspoon olive oil

1 clove garlic, crushed

3 cups low-sodium chicken stock

8 ounces escarole, washed and chopped, about 4 cups, firmly packed

1 tablespoon chopped parsley

¼ teaspoon dried basil

Salt and fresh ground black pepper to taste

1   Warm the oil in a 1½- to 2-quart saucepan over medium heat. Add the garlic and sauté 30 seconds until golden.

2   Add the stock, escarole, parsley, and basil. Raise the heat to high and bring to a boil. Reduce the heat to medium-low and simmer 5 to 7 minutes, until the escarole is tender.

3   Add the turkey meatballs to the soup. Simmer for 1 to 2 minutes, then season with salt and pepper. Serve hot.

PER SERVING:

212 calories	31 g protein	11 g total carbohydrates	4 g fiber	7 g net carbohydrates

5 Squares Classic
Split-Pea Soup

LEFTOVERS FREEZE BEAUTIFULLY FOR UP TO 3 MONTHS.

1 cup green split peas, soaked 6 to 8 hours in 1 quart water

5 cups low-sodium chicken stock

2 ounces Canadian bacon, finely chopped

1 small onion, peeled and finely chopped

1 small carrot, peeled and finely chopped

1 stalk celery, finely chopped

2 cloves garlic, crushed

1 bay leaf

Salt and fresh ground black pepper to taste

2 teaspoons chopped parsley

1   Drain the peas and place them in a heavy 2- to 3-quart saucepan.

2   Add 4 cups of stock and bring to a boil over high heat. Skim off and discard any fat that rises to the surface.

3   Add the bacon, onion, carrot, celery, garlic, and bay leaf.

4   Reduce the heat to low, add the remaining stock, and simmer covered for 1½ hours, stirring occasionally.

5   Season with salt and pepper. Discard the bay leaf and serve the soup piping hot, garnished with the chopped parsley.

PER SERVING:

308 calories	32 g protein	68 g total carbohydrates	25 g fiber	43 g net carbohydrates

Balsamic Marinated Chicken Strips with Mixed Greens

SERVES 2

6 ounces uncooked skinless boneless chicken breast

1½ tablespoons sugar-free balsamic dressing, plus additional to taste

3 cups mixed salad greens, such as spring mix or any combination of lettuces

1 Trim the chicken of any visible fat and slice into ½ inch-wide-strips. Toss with the sugar-free balsamic dressing.

2 Lightly spray a medium nonstick skillet with Pam and place it over medium heat. Add the chicken and sauté 3 to 4 minutes, stirring occasionally, until cooked through.

3 Toss the greens with additional dressing and mound it on plates. Top the greens with the chicken and serve.

PER SERVING:

82.5 calories	19.5 g protein	1.75 g total carbohydrates	1 g fiber	0.75 g net carbohydrates

Waldorf Chicken Salad with Raspberry Vinaigrette

6 ounces uncooked skinless boneless chicken breast

1 tablespoon Nayonaise

1 tablespoon spicy brown or Dijon mustard

2 teaspoons apple cider vinegar

¼ teaspoon Splenda (sugar-free sweetener)

2 tablespoons chopped celery

2 tablespoons chopped water chestnuts

½ apple, peeled and diced, about ¼ cup

Salt and fresh ground black pepper to taste

1 heart of romaine, roughly chopped, about 4 cups

6 cherry tomatoes, halved

1 small carrot, peeled and sliced into thin curls with a wide peeler

Sugar-free raspberry dressing to taste

¼ cup sliced or slivered almonds, lightly toasted (see Note)

1   Place the chicken in a saucepan and add enough water to cover. Steam covered on high for 10 to 12 minutes until cooked through.

2   Transfer the chicken to a plate and refrigerate until cool enough to handle.

3   In a large bowl combine the Nayonaise, mustard, vinegar, and Splenda. Whisk until smooth.

4   Add the celery, water chestnuts, and apple to the bowl.

5   Dice the chicken and add it to the bowl. Toss well and season with salt and pepper.

6   Toss the lettuce, tomatoes, and carrot ribbons with raspberry dressing. Divide on plates and top with the chicken salad. Sprinkle with the toasted almonds and serve.

NOTE: To toast the almonds, preheat the oven to 375°F. Spread the sliced or slivered almonds on a baking sheet and toast for 8 minutes until golden brown. Transfer to a plate to cool.

PER SERVING:

263 calories	26 g protein	18.6 g total carbohydrates	5.3 g fiber	13.3 g net carbohydrates

Roasted Garlic, Zucchini, and Chicken Soup

SERVES 2

1 head garlic

3 cups low-sodium chicken stock

3 ounces uncooked skinless boneless chicken breast, sliced into ½-inch-wide pieces

1 small zucchini, thinly sliced, about 1 cup

1 teaspoon chopped parsley

Salt and fresh ground black pepper to taste

1   Preheat the oven to 375°F.

2   Slice the garlic in half crosswise and lightly spray with Pam. Put the halves back together and wrap in foil. Bake for 45 minutes until soft.

3   Unwrap the garlic and set aside until it is cool enough to handle. Squeeze the garlic out of its skin into a small bowl and mash with a fork to a smooth paste.

4   Pour the chicken stock into a 1½- to 2-quart saucepan and bring to a boil over high heat. Reduce the heat to a simmer. Thin the roasted garlic paste with a little of the hot stock and add it to the pan.

5   Add the zucchini and chicken, and simmer for 10 to 15 minutes until the chicken is cooked through.

6   Add the parsley and season with salt and pepper. Serve piping hot.

PER SERVING:

117 calories	32 g protein	10 g total carbohydrates	1 g fiber	9 g net carbohydrates

Pasta Fagiole

SERVES 4

1 teaspoon olive oil

½ cup chopped onion

½ cup chopped carrots

½ cup chopped celery

½ clove garlic, crushed

½ teaspoon dried oregano

Pinch of red pepper flakes

One 14-ounce can low-sodium chicken stock

One 14-ounce can diced tomatoes with their juice

½ cup water, plus more if needed

½ cup brown rice elbow noodles (or any short pasta)

½ 14-ounce can kidney or pinto beans, rinsed and drained

3 to 4 fresh basil leaves, coarsely chopped

Salt

1   Heat the oil in a 1½- to 2-quart saucepan over medium heat. Add the onion, carrots, celery, garlic, oregano, and red pepper flakes and sauté 5 minutes until the vegetables soften.

2   Add the stock, the tomatoes and their juice, and water. Raise the heat and bring to a boil. Reduce the heat to low and simmer 10 minutes.

3   While the soup simmers, cook the pasta in a separate pan in 1 quart of lightly salted boiling water for 8 to 10 minutes until al dente. Drain the pasta. Stir the pasta and beans into the soup.

4   Add the basil and simmer 3 minutes. Season with salt. Thin the soup with a little water if it appears too thick. Serve immediately.

PER SERVING:

| 96.4 calories | 4.6 g protein | 21.4 g total carbohydrates | 4.8 g fiber | 16.6 g net carbohydrates |

Mushroom, Beef, and Barley Soup

SERVES 4

One 14-ounce can low-sodium beef broth

One 14-ounce can low-sodium chicken broth

¼ cup pearl barley

1 cup thinly sliced mushrooms

½ cup chopped onion

½ cup chopped carrots

½ cup chopped celery

1 bay leaf

1 teaspoon olive oil

6 ounces lean beef steak, diced

⅓ cup water

1 tablespoon chopped parsley

Salt and fresh ground black pepper to taste

1   In a 1½- to 2-quart saucepan combine the beef and chicken broths. Place the pan over high heat and bring to a boil.

2   Add the barley, mushrooms, onion, carrots, celery, and bay leaf. Reduce the heat to a simmer.

3   Meanwhile heat the oil in an 8-inch nonstick skillet over high heat until hot. Add the beef. Sear the meat on all sides for 2 to 3 minutes until well browned. Carefully add the water and scrape up any browned bits stuck to the bottom of the skillet. Transfer the beef and liquid into the soup pan.

4   Simmer the soup for 35 to 40 minutes until the barley is tender. Stir in the parsley, season with salt and pepper. Remove and discard the bay leaf before serving.

PER SERVING:

329 calories	34 g protein	20 g total carbohydrates	6 g fiber	14 g net carbohydrates

Perfect Shrimp Cocktail

8 ounces frozen or raw peeled shrimp (16 to 20 count)

4 ounces sugar-free cocktail sauce (such as Walden Farms)

1 lemon, cut into wedges

1   Bring to a boil 1 quart water with 1 teaspoon salt.

2   Add the shrimp (they can be still frozen) to the boiling water and cook 4 to 5 minutes until cooked through.

3   Drain and chill the shrimp under cold running water. Pat dry and serve with the cocktail sauce and lemon wedges.

PER SERVING:

131 calories	24 g protein	7 g total carbohydrates	3 g fiber	4 g net carbohydrates

Shrimp and
White Bean Salad

8 ounces raw shrimp, peeled and deveined

1 cup undrained canned white beans

1½ tablespoons distilled white vinegar

1 teaspoon olive oil

Pinch of red pepper flakes (optional)

⅛ teaspoon dried oregano

1 tablespoon chopped cilantro

Salt and fresh ground black pepper to taste

2 cups packaged mesclun greens

½ lemon, cut into wedges

1   Steam the shrimp over ½ inch of boiling water in a covered pan until cooked through (5–7 minutes, depending on size). Cool under cold running water. Drain well and transfer to a large bowl.

2   Drain the beans, reserving 1 tablespoon of their juice. Rinse them under cold running water and drain well. Transfer the beans to the bowl of shrimp.

3   Stir in the vinegar, oil, red pepper flakes, oregano, and cilantro. Toss with the reserved bean juice if the salad appears dry. Season with salt and pepper.

4   Serve the shrimp salad over the mesclun greens garnished with the lemon wedges.

PER SERVING:

| 270 calories | 32 g protein | 26 g total carbohydrates | 7 g fiber | 19 g net carbohydrates |

Chicken Salad with Cucumbers, Tomato, and Basil

6 ounces uncooked skinless boneless chicken breast

1 medium cucumber, peeled and diced, about 1 cup

1 small tomato, cored, seeded, and diced, about ½ cup

2 teaspoons distilled white vinegar

⅛ teaspoon Splenda (sugar-free sweetener)

1 teaspoon olive oil

2 tablespoons chopped fresh basil

Salt and fresh ground black pepper to taste

1. Bring to a boil 1 quart lightly salted water in a 1½- to 2-quart saucepan. Add the chicken and simmer covered for 8 to 10 minutes until cooked through. Drain and cool under cold running water. Pat dry and slice into ½-inch cubes.

2. Transfer the chicken to a mixing bowl. Add the cucumber, tomatoes, vinegar, Splenda, olive oil, and basil. Season with salt and pepper and toss to combine.

PER SERVING:

193 calories	28 g protein	6 g total carbohydrates	3 g fiber	3 g net carbohydrates

5 Squares Tuna Salad

SERVES 2

12 ounces chunk light tuna packed in water

¼ cup chopped carrot

¼ cup chopped celery

2 tablespoons chopped water chestnuts

¼ cup plus 1 teaspoon Nayonaise

1 teaspoon prepared mustard

1 teaspoon distilled white vinegar

½ teaspoon lemon juice

Salt and fresh ground black pepper to taste

1 small cucumber, peeled and thinly sliced

1 small carrot, peeled into long curls

4 cherry tomatoes, halved

1 Drain the tuna in a sieve. Rinse it under cold running water and squeeze out any excess water. Transfer the tuna to a medium bowl.

2 Add the carrot, celery, water chestnuts, Nayonaise, mustard, vinegar, and lemon juice. Toss to combine. Season with salt and pepper and toss again.

3 Serve the salad garnished with sliced cucumber, carrot curls, and cherry tomatoes.

PER SERVING:

308 calories	44.3 g protein	15 g total carbohydrates	1.4 g fiber	13.6 g net carbohydrates

Turkey Salad with Chopped Apple, Tomato, and Romaine

SERVES 2

8 ounces fresh roasted turkey breast, chopped, about 2 cups

1 apple, peeled and chopped

1 plum tomato, chopped

½ tablespoon yellow mustard

2 tablespoons Nayonaise

⅛ teaspoon Splenda (sugar-free sweetener)

Salt and fresh ground black pepper to taste

2 hearts of romaine, chopped, about 4 cups

1 small carrot, peeled into long curls

1 small cucumber, peeled and thinly sliced

1 In a mixing bowl, combine the turkey, apple, tomato, mustard, Nayonaise, and Splenda. Season with salt and pepper and mix well.

2 Divide the romaine on two plates. Mound the turkey salad over the romaine and garnish with carrot curls and cucumber slices.

PER SERVING:

288 calories	37.5 g protein	19 g total carbohydrates	4.5 g fiber	14.5 g net carbohydrates

Fresh Crabmeat Salad

2 tablespoons fresh lemon juice

1 tablespoon distilled white vinegar

½ teaspoon salt

⅛ teaspoon cayenne pepper

1 tablespoon chopped fresh dill

1 teaspoon olive oil

8 ounces fresh lump crabmeat

1 small cucumber, peeled, seeded, and diced, about ½ cup

1 tablespoon minced red onion

1   In a medium bowl whisk the lemon juice, vinegar, salt, cayenne, dill, and olive oil.

2   Discard any cartilage from the crabmeat. Transfer to the bowl of dressing and toss. Fold in the cucumbers and red onion and serve.

PER SERVING:

114 calories	14 g protein	3 g total carbohydrates	1 g fiber	2 g net carbohydrates

Zesty Grilled Marinated Chicken Salad

6 ounces uncooked skinless boneless chicken breast

3 tablespoons sugar-free Italian dressing

4 cups prewashed packaged baby spinach

Sugar-free raspberry dressing to taste

2 large strawberries, thinly sliced, or ½ cup fresh raspberries

1 Preheat the oven to 375°F.

2 Trim any visible fat from the chicken and toss with sugar-free Italian dressing. Refrigerate for 1 hour or overnight.

3 Lightly spray a grill pan with Pam and place over medium heat. When the pan is hot, add the chicken and grill 2 minutes per side. Transfer the grill pan to the oven and bake 8 to 10 minutes until the chicken is cooked through.

4 Transfer the chicken to a cutting surface to cool. Slice it into thin strips.

5 In a large bowl toss the spinach with the raspberry dressing.

6 Mound the spinach onto two plates. Top each plate with the chicken. Garnish with the sliced strawberries or raspberries.

PER SERVING:

102 calories	20.4 g protein	3.6 g total carbohydrates	2.5 g fiber	1.1 g net carbohydrates

Lentil Turkey Salad with Green Beans

3 cups cold water

⅓ cup lentils

1 bay leaf

1 cup green beans, sliced into ½-inch pieces

6 ounces fresh roasted turkey breast, chopped

1 plum tomato, cored and diced

1 tablespoon chopped fresh dill

1 scallion, thinly sliced

1 tablespoon Nayonaise

1 tablespoon lemon juice

Salt and fresh ground black pepper to taste

1   Combine the cold water, lentils, and bay leaf in a 2-quart saucepan and bring to a boil over high heat. Reduce the heat to low and simmer 20 minutes until the lentils are tender but not falling apart. Drain in a sieve, discard the bay leaf, and spread on a plate to cool.

2   Steam the green beans over ½ inch of boiling water in a covered pan for 2 to 3 minutes until bright green and tender. Drain the beans and cool under cold running water. Pat dry and transfer to a large mixing bowl.

3   Add the turkey, lentils, tomato, dill, and scallions to the green beans.

4   Stir in the Nayonaise and lemon juice. Season with salt and pepper and serve.

PER SERVING:

229 calories	30 g protein	14 g total carbohydrates	3 g fiber	11 g net carbohydrates

Steamed Salmon Fillet over Mesclun Greens

Two 4-ounce salmon fillets

Salt and fresh ground black pepper to taste

2 tablespoons chopped fresh dill

4 cups mesclun greens

2 to 3 tablespoons sugar-free honey-mustard vinaigrette

Lemon wedges for garnish

1   Season the fillets with salt and pepper. Press the dill into the flesh.

2   Steam the salmon over ½ inch of boiling water in a covered pan for 8 to 10 minutes until cooked through. Transfer to a plate.

3   In a bowl toss the greens with the dressing and mound on two plates. Top the greens with the salmon and serve garnished with the lemon wedges.

PER SERVING:

122 calories	13 g protein	4 g total carbohydrates	1 g fiber	3 g net carbohydrates

Barbecue Grilled Chicken with Sweet and Sour Cucumbers

SERVES 2

6 ounces uncooked skinless boneless chicken breast

2 tablespoons sugar-free barbecue sauce

1   Toss the chicken breast with the barbecue sauce and refrigerate at least 1 hour or overnight.

2   Heat a grill pan over medium heat until hot. Grill the chicken 4 to 5 minutes per side until cooked through. Transfer the chicken to a cutting surface to cool. Slice into thin strips. Serve over Sweet and Sour Cucumbers (below).

SWEET AND SOUR CUCUMBERS

1 large or 2 small cucumbers, peeled and thinly sliced, about 2 cups

1 small carrot, peeled and coarsely grated, about 1/3 cup

1/2 teaspoon salt

2 tablespoons distilled white vinegar

1/4 teaspoon Splenda (sugar-free sweetener)

Fresh ground black pepper to taste

Combine the cucumbers and carrots in a bowl; toss with salt, vinegar, and Splenda. Season with black pepper and serve as directed above.

PER SERVING:

113 calories	24 g protein	6 g total carbohydrates	2 g fiber	4 g net carbohydrates

Spicy Lime and Cumin–Marinated Chicken with Spinach

SERVES 2

Juice of 1 lime

1 teaspoon ground cumin

¼ teaspoon paprika

⅛ teaspoon cayenne pepper

½ teaspoon salt

1 clove garlic, crushed

1 teaspoon olive oil

6 ounces uncooked skinless boneless chicken breast

4 cups packaged prewashed baby spinach

2 tablespoons sugar-free balsamic dressing or to taste

3 cherry tomatoes, halved

1 In a medium bowl whisk to combine the lime juice, cumin, paprika, cayenne pepper, salt, garlic, and olive oil.

2 Slice the chicken into ½-inch strips, add them to the bowl with the marinade, and toss to coat. Refrigerate for 1 hour.

3 Heat a grill pan over medium heat until hot. Grill the chicken 3 to 4 minutes per side until cooked through.

4 Toss the spinach with the dressing. Serve the chicken over the spinach, garnished with the cherry tomatoes.

PER SERVING:

149 calories	21 g protein	8 g total carbohydrates	5 g fiber	3 g net carbohydrates

Fresh Salmon Salad with Capers and Dill

8 ounces salmon fillet, skinned

½ cup Nayonaise

1 tablespoon fresh lemon juice

⅛ teaspoon Splenda (sugar-free sweetener)

1 stalk celery, finely diced, about ⅓ cup

1 tablespoon chopped fresh dill

1 teaspoon capers, drained

Salt and fresh ground black pepper to taste

4 cups prewashed spring mix or 1 romaine heart, chopped

2 tablespoons sugar-free balsamic dressing or to taste

1   Steam the salmon over ½ inch of boiling water in a covered pan for 8 minutes until cooked through. Transfer the salmon to a plate and break up with a fork. Refrigerate until cool.

2   Transfer the salmon to a bowl and stir in the Nayonaise, lemon juice, Splenda, celery, dill, and capers. Season with salt and pepper.

3   Toss the greens or chopped romaine with the dressing and divide between two plates. Mound the salmon salad over the greens and serve.

PER SERVING:

371 calories	28 g protein	8.4 g total carbohydrates	2 g fiber	6.4 g net carbohydrates

Fresh Whitefish Salad with Cucumbers and Red Onion Vinaigrette

SERVES 2

1 small red onion, diced, about ¼ cup

1 tablespoon rice vinegar

1 tablespoon fresh lemon juice

⅛ teaspoon Splenda (sugar-free sweetener)

¼ teaspoon salt

8 ounces red snapper fillet, skinless

1 tablespoon olive oil

1 small cucumber, peeled and diced, about ½ cup

1 plum tomato, diced

1 tablespoon chopped cilantro or parsley

Fresh ground black pepper to taste

1   Combine diced onion, rice vinegar, lemon juice, Splenda, and salt in a bowl and refrigerate 30 minutes.

2   Steam the snapper over ½ inch of boiling water in a covered pan for 7 to 8 minutes until cooked through. Transfer the fish to a plate and break up with a fork. Refrigerate until cool.

3   Transfer the fish to the chilled marinade. Add the olive oil, cucumber, tomato, and cilantro or parsley and toss to combine. Season with salt and pepper. Toss again and serve.

PER SERVING:

152 calories	24 g protein	4 g total carbohydrates	1 g fiber	3 g net carbohydrates

DANA SINGER'S 5 SQUARES
MAKEOVER SUCCESS STORY

I HEARD ABOUT 5 SQUARES FROM a friend. It sounded like a good idea; but I waited a month before I actually took the plunge. I was on the verge of turning 32. I realized that the weight I had put on in the past 7 years was problematic. After all, my mother, who has since passed away, was diagnosed with Type II (Adult Onset) Diabetes at an age a little beyond the one I was approaching. The doctors told her that her weight had a great deal to do with the onset of the diabetes. Furthermore, she was the second generation to receive this diagnosis. I knew fairly well that diabetes is typically genetic, and this concerned me greatly.

In 1998, I moved from my native Los Angeles to Connecticut. Before I left, I requested that my doctors give me copies of my medical history, so I could find appropriate treatment in my new home base. I was curious enough to look at the records. As I read through the first three or four, I was shocked to find that each record characterized me as a 28-year-old Caucasian female who was "obese." When I saw that word over and over, I had to reexamine my own feelings about myself. The characterization came as both a shock and a terrible blow. I had a great deal of trouble absorbing the truth.

Weight problems also ran in my family. Both my parents were always overweight by at least 60 to 90 pounds. As I thought about starting on the 5 squares meal plan, I realized that I had never learned how to eat properly and healthfully. We ate out often or my dad grilled some kind of beef while my mother baked potatoes we would smother in butter, sour cream, and sometimes cheese. Then, she would use the microwave to heat up a hearty Stouffer's side dish like escalloped apples, creamed spinach, spinach soufflé, or my dad's favorite—noodles Romanoff. When I think of the eating habits I adopted as a child, it is no wonder I ended up where I did. Not to mention that exercise has always been a four-letter word in my family.

Ultimately, however, I decided to get healthy. On July 29, 2002, I received my first delivery from 5 squares. The food was wonderful. It filled me up. The 5 squares staff told me that I was welcome to have a homemade salad with any meal, provided I did not use any vegetables that were considered carbohydrates. I never needed to supplement because there was always plenty to eat. In fact, as my weight loss progressed, the meals became too much to eat in one sitting.

I found myself losing 10 to 13 pounds per month. This plan really gets your metabolism moving, so you burn calories no matter what you do. And others noticed the change in me too. One day my husband came over to hug me, and said, "It is so nice to hug you and actually be able to get my arms all the way around you!" I was stunned! I had never realized he couldn't do so before.

I have now adopted a new nutritional lifestyle, one in which I can eat a tasty variety of foods, but control my portions and keep the carbs low. My last meal delivery was December 17, 2003—less than 5 months since I'd begun the program. My total weight loss was 60 pounds. I can wear clothes I have not worn since college. It feels great. And I must admit to enjoying the praise I hear from friends and family when we see each other.

On a last note, I promise that you can follow this diet and do all the cooking yourself. Since my last meal delivery, I have lost an additional 8 pounds—even with occasional cheating. All you have to do is follow the recipes, follow the time schedule, read labels at the grocery store, and make sure to stay aware and educated about what you're eating.

5 squares has made me set new standards with a lifestyle that works and that I can readily follow.

Turkey Meatballs à la Marinara with Brown Rice Ziti

SERVES 2

FOR THE TURKEY MEATBALLS:

12 ounces ground turkey

1 large egg, lightly beaten

2 teaspoons finely chopped parsley

1 teaspoon oregano

2 tablespoons quick oats

4 tablespoons sugar-free marinara sauce

1 teaspoon olive oil

2 tablespoons finely chopped onion

2 cloves garlic, crushed

Pinch of salt

Fresh ground black pepper to taste

2 cups sugar-free marinara sauce

1 cup, cooked, brown rice ziti

1   Preheat the oven to 375°F.

2   In a large bowl combine the turkey, egg, parsley, oregano, oats, and 4 tablespoons marinara sauce.

3   Warm the oil in a small sauté pan over medium heat. Add the onion, garlic, and a pinch of salt. Sauté for 2 to 3 minutes until lightly browned. Transfer the sautéed onion and garlic to the turkey mixture in the bowl and mix well. Season with salt and pepper.

4   Form the turkey mixture into six balls and transfer to a 6 by 8-inch baking pan or pie plate. Lightly spray with Pam and bake for 20 minutes until cooked through.

5   Heat 2 cups marinara sauce in a pan over medium heat until hot. Add the turkey balls and cook 1 minute.

6   Serve over brown rice ziti.

| 381 calories | 337.3 g protein | 7.4 g total carbohydrates | 1.5 g fiber | 5.9 g net carbohydrates |

Lemon-Garlic Chicken with Rosemary-Roasted Potatoes and Sautéed String Beans Almandine

SERVES 2

3 cloves garlic, crushed

1 teaspoon McCormick Lemon & Pepper Seasoning Salt

2 tablespoons fresh lemon juice

1 teaspoon olive oil

2 whole uncooked skinless boneless chicken breasts, about 6 ounces each

Salt and fresh ground black pepper to taste

2 thin rounds of sliced lemon

½ teaspoon paprika

1   Preheat the oven to 375°F. Lightly spray a 6 by 8-inch baking pan with Pam.

2   In a medium bowl mix the garlic, lemon pepper seasoning, lemon juice, and olive oil.

3   Add the chicken and toss to coat. Season with salt and pepper.

4   Transfer the chicken to the baking pan, smooth side up. Lay a lemon slice on each breast half, dust with paprika. Lightly spray the chicken with Pam.

5   Bake for 20 to 25 minutes until cooked through. Serve with Rosemary-Roasted Potatoes and Sautéed String Beans Almandine (page 91).

ROSEMARY-ROASTED POTATOES

2 medium red potatoes, about 4 ounces each, quartered

1 teaspoon chopped fresh rosemary or ½ teaspoon dried rosemary

1 teaspoon olive oil

Salt and fresh ground black pepper to taste

1   Preheat the oven to 375°F. Lightly spray a pie plate with Pam.

2   Toss the potato wedges with the rosemary, olive oil, salt, and pepper. Place them in the pie plate and roast for 25 minutes or until tender.

SAUTÉED STRING BEANS ALMANDINE

½ teaspoon olive oil

6 ounces haricots verts (slender French green beans), fresh or frozen

Small pinch of red pepper flakes

2 tablespoons low-sodium chicken stock

1 tablespoon sliced almonds, lightly toasted (page 67)

Warm the oil in a small nonstick skillet over high heat. Add the haricots, pepper flakes, and chicken stock. Sauté for 2 to 3 minutes, stirring often until bright green and tender. Toss with the almonds and serve.

PER SERVING:

259 calories	31 g protein	25 g total carbohydrates	5 g fiber	20 g net carbohydrates

Stuffed Flank Steak with Spinach and Onions over Seasoned Barley

SERVES 4

FOR THE STEAK:

16 ounces flank steak, butterflied

1 teaspoon olive oil

Salt and fresh ground black pepper to taste

2 tablespoons chopped fresh basil

1 tablespoon chopped fresh parsley

1 teaspoon chopped fresh rosemary

2 cloves garlic, minced

FOR THE STUFFING:

1 teaspoon olive oil

16 ounces packed baby spinach

2 tablespoons low-sodium chicken stock

1 cup thinly sliced onion

Salt and fresh ground pepper to taste

1   Rub the steak with oil and season with salt and pepper. Sprinkle both sides with the chopped herbs and garlic. Refrigerate for 2 hours or overnight.

2   To make the stuffing: heat the oil in a 10- to 12-inch-wide nonstick skillet over high heat. Add the spinach and stock and cook for 1 to 2 minutes until the spinach is wilted. Transfer the spinach to a bowl and drain the juices back into the pan.

3   Add the onion to the pan and sauté over medium heat for 2 to 3 minutes until softened and lightly browned.

4   Transfer the onion to the spinach and mix well. Season with salt and pepper.

5   Lightly spray a 6 by 8-inch baking pan with Pam. Lay the steak on the pan. Spread the spinach mixture evenly over the steak leaving a ½-inch border all around. Roll up the steak and position it seam side down.

6   Roast the steak for 25 to 30 minutes for medium-rare.

7   Let the steak rest, loosely covered with foil, for 10 minutes before slicing.

8   Serve the steak over the Seasoned Barley, drizzled with the pan juices.

SEASONED BARLEY

⅓ cup pearl barley

2 cups low-sodium chicken stock

1 cup water

1 teaspoon McCormick Lemon & Pepper Seasoning Salt

1 slice lemon, seeds removed

2 teaspoons finely chopped fresh parsley

Salt to taste

1   Combine the barley, stock, water, lemon pepper seasoning, and lemon slice in a 1- to 2-quart saucepan and bring to a boil over high heat. Reduce the heat to low and simmer covered for 30 minutes until the barley is tender.

2   Drain the barley and toss with the parsley. Season with salt and serve.

PER SERVING:

| 366 calories | 27 g protein | 25 g total carbohydrates | 4.7 g fiber | 20.3 g net carbohydrates |

Chicken Piccata with Steamed Asparagus and Savory Mushroom Brown Rice

12 ounces uncooked skinless boneless chicken breasts, halved

Salt and fresh ground black pepper to taste

½ cup cornstarch

⅓ cup egg whites

1 tablespoon lemon juice

½ cup low-sodium chicken stock

1 tablespoon capers, drained

2 teaspoons chopped fresh parsley

8 plump asparagus spears, washed and trimmed

1   Season the chicken with the salt and pepper.

2   Lightly spray a 10- to 12-inch nonstick skillet with Pam and place over medium heat.

3   Spread the cornstarch on a plate. Place the egg whites in a shallow bowl.

4   Dredge the chicken halves in cornstarch and then dip them in the egg whites.

5   Sauté the chicken 3 minutes per side until golden brown.

6   Add the lemon juice, stock, capers, and parsley to the pan and simmer covered over medium heat for 7 to 8 minutes until cooked through.

7   Lay the asparagus in a steamer insert and place them in a frying pan or saucepan. Pour in about 1 inch of boiling water, then season with salt and cover. Steam them for 5 to 6 minutes or until they feel tender when tested with a skewer.

8   Serve over Savory Mushroom Brown Rice with Steamed Asparagus on the side.

SAVORY MUSHROOM BROWN RICE

SERVES 6 (½ CUP PER SERVING, COOKED)

1 teaspoon olive oil

2 ounces button mushrooms, thinly sliced, about 1 cup

1 cup long-grain brown rice

2 cups low-sodium chicken stock

1 teaspoon chopped fresh parsley

2 teaspoons chopped fresh cilantro

1   Warm the oil in a heavy 1- to 2-quart saucepan over medium heat. Add the mushrooms and sauté 2 to 3 minutes until lightly browned. Stir in the rice and sauté 1 minute.

2   Add the stock, parsley, and cilantro and bring to a boil. Reduce the heat to low and simmer covered for 40 minutes or until the rice is tender and all the liquid has been absorbed.

PER SERVING:

283 calories	74 g protein	18 g total carbohydrates	4 g fiber	14 g net carbohydrates

Turkey Meatloaf with Sautéed Spinach and 5 Squares Mashed Potatoes

SERVES 2

1 small carrot, peeled and halved lengthwise

1 small stalk celery, trimmed and halved lengthwise

1 recipe Turkey Meatballs (page 88), uncooked

¼ teaspoon dried oregano

1 cup canned crushed tomato

2 leaves fresh basil

1 recipe Sautéed Spinach (page 105)

1 Preheat the oven to 375°F. Lightly spray a 6 by 8-inch baking pan with Pam.

2 Steam the carrot and celery over ½ inch of boiling water in a covered pan for 5 minutes until tender.

3 Place the turkey mixture in the baking pan and form into a six-inch loaf.

4 Form 2 lengthwise indentations large enough to hold the carrot and celery pieces. Lay the carrot and celery in place and fold the sides of the loaf over them to conceal them.

5 Smooth the loaf and sprinkle it with oregano. Pour the tomatoes over the loaf, tear the basil leaves, and sprinkle them over all.

6 Cover the pan with aluminum foil and bake 20 minutes. Uncover and bake 5 minutes more until browned. Serve with Sautéed Spinach and 5 Squares Mashed Potatoes (page 97).

5 SQUARES MASHED POTATOES

1 Idaho potato, about 8 ounces, peeled and quartered

3 to 4 tablespoons low-sodium chicken stock, at room temperature

Salt and fresh ground pepper to taste

1 Place the potato in a small saucepan and cover with cold water. Bring to a boil, reduce the heat to low, and simmer 15 minutes until tender.

2 Drain the potato and return it to the pan. Add the chicken stock and mash to desired consistency. Season with salt and pepper.

PER SERVING:

316 calories	39 g protein	27 g total carbohydrates	3 g fiber	24 g net carbohydrates

Mustard-Baked Swordfish with Quick Tomato Salsa and Steamed Broccoli

SERVES 2

2 swordfish steaks, 1 inch thick, about 6 ounces each

2 tablespoons prepared spicy brown mustard or grainy Dijon

QUICK TOMATO SALSA:

1 large tomato, diced, about 1 cup

1 small onion, diced, about ⅓ cup

2 tablespoons chopped fresh basil

1 teaspoon olive oil

Salt and fresh ground black pepper to taste

2 cups broccoli florets

Lemon wedges for serving

1   Preheat the oven to 375°F. Lightly spray a 6 by 8-inch baking pan with Pam.

2   Slather the swordfish with the mustard and place it in the pan. Bake 15 minutes until cooked through.

3   Meanwhile, in a bowl, combine the tomato, onion, basil, and oil. Season with salt and pepper and toss well.

4   Steam the broccoli over ½ inch of boiling water in a covered pan for 3 to 4 minutes until tender.

5   Serve the fish topped with salsa, with the broccoli and lemon wedges on the side.

PER SERVING:

199 calories	25 g protein	18 g total carbohydrates	2 g fiber	16 g net carbohydrates

Beef Stir-Fry

SERVES 2

½ tablespoon wheat-free tamari soy sauce, plus additional to taste

½ teaspoon minced fresh ginger

1 small clove garlic, crushed

1 tablespoon fresh lime juice

⅛ teaspoon Splenda (sugar-free sweetener)

8 ounces sirloin steak, thinly sliced

FOR THE STIR-FRY:

2 teaspoons vegetable oil

½ teaspoon minced fresh ginger

Small pinch of red pepper flakes (optional)

1 cup red cabbage, sliced into ¼-inch strips

1 cup carrots, peeled and sliced into ¼-inch strips

½ red bell pepper, cored and sliced into ¼-inch strips

½ cup sliced water chestnuts

10 pieces canned baby corn

2 tablespoons chopped fresh cilantro

1   Combine the tamari, ginger, garlic, lime juice, and Splenda in a bowl. Add the beef strips and toss to coat. Cover and refrigerate for 2 hours or overnight.

2   In a wok or wide nonstick skillet over high heat combine the oil, ginger, and red pepper flakes, if using, and sizzle for 10 to 15 seconds.

3   Add the cabbage, carrots, pepper, water chestnuts, and baby corn. Stir-fry 3 to 4 minutes until the vegetables begin to soften.

4   Add the beef with its marinade to the wok and stir fry 3 to 4 minutes until the beef is cooked through. Season with more tamari and stir in the cilantro. Serve immediately.

PER SERVING:

252 calories	23.55 g protein	22 g total carbohydrates	2.5 g fiber	19.5 g net carbohydrates

Stuffed Peppers with Herbed Tomato Sauce and Braised Cabbage

SERVES 2

FOR THE STUFFED PEPPERS:

1 recipe Turkey Meatballs, uncooked (page 88)

1 tablespoon chopped raisins

1 large red bell pepper, halved, seeded, and cored

FOR THE TOMATO SAUCE:

2 cups canned tomato puree

4 tablespoons finely diced onion

2 tablespoons finely diced celery

1 clove garlic, crushed to a paste

1 tablespoon chopped fresh basil

1 tablespoon chopped fresh parsley

Salt and fresh ground black pepper to taste

1   Preheat the oven to 375°F.

2   Toss the prepared turkey filling with the raisins. Refrigerate while you make the sauce.

3   Combine all of the sauce ingredients in a medium saucepan and simmer over low heat for 10 minutes. Transfer the sauce to a 6 by 8-inch baking dish.

4   Stuff the pepper halves with the turkey filling and place them over the sauce.

5   Bake for 20 minutes until cooked through. Serve over Braised Cabbage (page 101).

BRAISED CABBAGE

1 teaspoon olive oil

1 cup red cabbage, sliced into ¼-inch strips

2 cups green cabbage, sliced into ¼-inch strips

Pinch of salt

½ cup low-sodium chicken stock

1 tablespoon distilled white vinegar

Fresh ground black pepper to taste

1 In a medium sauté pan over high heat, add the oil and cabbages, and a pinch of salt. Sauté 2 minutes stirring frequently until the cabbage begins to soften.

2 Add the chicken stock and vinegar. Reduce the heat to low and simmer covered for 10 to 12 minutes until the cabbage is tender. Season with salt and pepper.

PER SERVING:

426.4 calories	45 g protein	52 g total carbohydrates	4 g fiber	48 g net carbohydrates

Marinated Fajita with Garlic Sautéed Broccoli and Baked Sliced Sweet Potato

SERVES 2

FOR THE MARINADE:

½ cup fresh basil leaves

½ cup fresh parsley leaves

½ cup fresh cilantro leaves

2 tablespoons olive oil

¼ low-sodium chicken stock

½ teaspoon salt

¼ teaspoon fresh ground black pepper

1 clove garlic

¼ teaspoon red pepper flakes

One 8-ounce flank steak

1 recipe Baked Sliced Sweet Potato

1 recipe Garlic Sautéed Broccoli (page 149)

1   Combine the marinade ingredients in a blender and puree until smooth.

2   Transfer the marinade to a Ziploc bag. Add the steak and turn to coat with marinade. Refrigerate for 2 hours or overnight.

3   Place a grill pan over medium-high heat until hot. Grill the steak with its marinade 4 to 5 minutes per side for medium-rare. Transfer the steak to a cutting surface and cover loosely with foil. Let rest 5 minutes. Slice on an angle across the grain into thin strips. Serve fajitas over Baked Sliced Sweet Potato (page 103) with Garlic Sautéed Broccoli on the side.

BAKED SLICED SWEET POTATO

1 medium sweet potato, about 8 ounces

Salt and fresh ground black pepper to taste

1 teaspoon olive oil

1. Preheat the oven to 375°F. Lightly spray a 6 by 8-inch baking pan with Pam.

2. Slice the sweet potato into ½-inch-thick rounds.

3. Season the potato with salt and pepper and toss with the oil. Transfer to the baking pan and bake 25 to 30 minutes until tender. Turn the potato halfway through for even browning.

PER SERVING:

315 calories	26 g protein	28 g total carbohydrates	4 g fiber	24 g net carbohydrates

Baked Spice-Rubbed Salmon with Sautéed Spinach

SERVES 2

FOR THE SPICE RUB:

1 tablespoon lemon juice

1 teaspoon finely grated lemon zest

2 teaspoons chopped fresh dill

½ teaspoon salt

¼ teaspoon fresh ground black pepper

½ teaspoon granulated garlic or 1 teaspoon minced fresh garlic

2 fillets of salmon, about 4 to 5 ounces each, skin removed

Lemon wedges for garnish

1   Combine the ingredients for the Spice Rub and rub it into both sides of the salmon. Transfer the fish to a plate and wrap with plastic. Refrigerate up to 1 hour.

2   Preheat the oven to 425°F. Lightly spray a 6 by 8-inch baking pan with Pam.

3   Place the salmon in the pan and roast for 12 minutes for medium-rare.

4   Serve the salmon over Sautéed Spinach (page 105) accompanied by the lemon wedges.

SAUTÉED SPINACH

1 teaspoon olive oil

½ teaspoon minced garlic (optional)

8 ounces prewashed baby spinach, about 2 cups

Salt and fresh ground black pepper to taste

In a 10- to 12-inch skillet over medium heat, add the oil, garlic, if using, and spinach and sauté stirring constantly for 2 to 3 minutes until the spinach wilts. Season with salt and pepper.

PER SERVING:

| 232 calories | 23 g protein | 3 g total carbohydrates | 1 g fiber | 2 g net carbohydrates |

Stuffed Eggplant with Mashed Sweet Potatoes

SERVES 2

1 medium purple eggplant, about 12 ounces

Salt and fresh ground black pepper to taste

1 recipe Turkey Meatballs, uncooked (page 88)

1   Preheat the oven to 375°F. Lightly spray a 6 by 8-inch baking pan with Pam.

2   Trim the eggplant and slice it lengthwise in half. Scoop out and discard the seeds and some of the pulp from the eggplant halves to form a cavity with a ½-inch border. Season lightly with salt and pepper.

3   Mound the turkey into the eggplant halves and then transfer them to the baking pan. Lightly spray the turkey with Pam.

4   Bake for 25 minutes until the eggplant is tender and the turkey is cooked through. Serve with Mashed Sweet Potatoes (below).

MASHED SWEET POTATOES

1 medium sweet potato, about 8 ounces, peeled and diced

Sugar-free maple syrup to taste (such as Maple Grove Farms Cozy Cottage)

Ground cinnamon to taste

1   Place the sweet potato in a 1- to 2-quart saucepan and cover with cold water. Bring to a boil over high heat.

2   Reduce the heat to low and simmer 15 minutes or until the potato is tender. Drain the potato and return it to the pan. Mash with the sugar-free syrup. Sprinkle with a little ground cinnamon and serve.

PER SERVING:

262 calories	34.5 g protein	14.7 g total carbohydrates	6.5 g fiber	8.2 g net carbohydrates

Shrimp à la Française with Sweet Peas and Carrots

½ cup cornstarch

⅓ cup egg whites

8 ounces large shrimp, peeled, deveined, and butterflied

¼ teaspoon cayenne pepper (optional)

2 tablespoons lemon juice

⅓ cup low-sodium chicken stock

1 tablespoon chopped fresh dill

Salt and fresh ground black pepper to taste

1 recipe Sweet Peas and Carrots (page 175)

1   Spread the cornstarch on a plate and place the egg whites in a shallow bowl.

2   Season the shrimp with cayenne, if using. Dredge the shrimp in the cornstarch and dip in the egg white. Transfer to a plate. Discard the remaining cornstarch.

3   Lightly spray an 8- or 10-inch nonstick skillet with Pam and place over high heat. Add the shrimp and sauté 2 minutes per side until golden brown.

4   Add the lemon juice, stock, and dill and simmer for 2 minutes until the shrimp are cooked through. Season with salt and pepper and serve with Sweet Peas and Carrots.

PER SERVING:

234.7 calories	28.75 g protein	21 g total carbohydrates	1.5 g fiber	19.5 g net carbohydrates

Roast Pork Loin with Fresh Herbs and Roasted Vegetables

SERVES 2

16 ounces pork loin, butterflied

1 teaspoon olive oil

Salt and fresh ground black pepper to taste

2 tablespoons chopped fresh basil

1 tablespoon chopped fresh parsley

2 teaspoons chopped fresh sage

2 cloves garlic, minced, plus 6 cloves garlic, peeled but left whole

2 cups low-sodium chicken stock

2 medium carrots, sliced into ½-inch pieces

1 large onion, peeled and coarsely chopped

1 stalk celery, sliced into ½-inch pieces

1 bay leaf

1   Preheat the oven to 350°F.

2   Rub the pork loin with the oil and season with salt and pepper. Lay the loin flat on a cutting surface, smooth side down. Spread the basil, parsley, sage, and minced garlic evenly over the surface of the pork and roll up.

3   Bring the chicken stock to a boil in a small saucepan. Pour the stock into a medium baking dish large enough to hold the pork with a little room to spare.

4   Spread the carrots, onion, celery, whole garlic, and bay leaf in the pan.

5   Place the rolled pork, seam side down, on top of the vegetables. Lightly spray the pork with Pam. Cover the pan with foil.

6   Roast the pork for 30 minutes. Uncover and roast 15 to 20 minutes until an

instant-read thermometer inserted into the center of the meat registers 140°F. Remove the pan from the oven and discard the bay leaf.

7   Let the roast rest, loosely covered with foil, for 10 minutes before slicing.

8   Serve the sliced pork with the vegetables and pan gravy.

PER SERVING:

| 170 calories | 20 g protein | 9.75 g total carbohydrates | 1 g fiber | 8.75 g net carbohydrates |

Sautéed Tilapia with Black Bean and Corn Salad and Sautéed Broccoli Rabe

SERVES 2

Two 6-ounce tilapia fillets

Salt and fresh ground black pepper to taste

Lemon wedges for garnish

1 recipe Sautéed Broccoli Rabe (page 155)

1   Preheat the oven to 400°F. Lightly spray a large ovenproof nonstick skillet with Pam. Season fillets with salt and pepper.

2   Heat the skillet over high heat until hot. Add the fillets and reduce the heat to medium. Sauté 2 minutes per side.

3   Transfer the pan to the oven and bake 5 to 7 minutes until cooked through.

4   Serve the fish, garnished with the lemon wedges, over Sautéed Broccoli Rabe with some Black Bean and Corn Salad (below) on the side.

BLACK BEAN AND CORN SALAD

SERVES 2–3

½ cup frozen corn kernels

1 cup drained and rinsed canned black beans

2 tablespoons diced red bell pepper

1 tablespoon chopped red onion (optional)

2 tablespoons chopped fresh cilantro or basil

1 tablespoon sugar-free balsamic dressing

1 tablespoon fresh lime juice

Salt and fresh ground black pepper to taste

1 Steam the corn over ½ inch of boiling water in a covered pan for 2 to 3 minutes until cooked through. Drain and cool under cold running water.

2 In a medium bowl toss the corn, beans, bell pepper, red onion, if using, cilantro or basil, balsamic dressing, and lime juice to combine. Season with salt and pepper.

PER SERVING:

270 calories	19 g protein	33 g total carbohydrates	9 g fiber	24 g net carbohydrates

Turkey Cutlets with Rosemary Gravy, Garlic Mashed Potatoes, and Sautéed Sugar Snap Peas

SERVES 2

12 ounces turkey cutlets (2 to 4 pieces per person, depending on size)

Salt and fresh ground black pepper to taste

FOR THE ROSEMARY GRAVY:

2 teaspoons cornstarch

1 cup low-sodium chicken stock

1 teaspoon wheat-free tamari soy sauce

1 branch fresh rosemary, about 4 to 6 inches

1 recipe Garlic Mashed Potatoes (page 151)

1 recipe Sautéed Sugar Snap Peas (page 179)

1   Season the turkey with salt and pepper. Lightly spray an 8- or 10-inch non-stick skillet with Pam and heat over high heat.

2   Add the turkey cutlets to the skillet and reduce the heat to medium. Sauté 3 to 4 minutes per side until cooked through. Remove cutlets to a plate.

3   To make the rosemary gravy, dissolve the cornstarch in 2 tablespoons of the chicken stock in a small bowl. Add the remaining stock and the soy sauce and mix well. Pour into the skillet. Add the rosemary and bring to a boil. Reduce the heat to low and simmer 1 minute until the sauce thickens. Return the turkey and any juices to the skillet for 1 to 2 minutes until heated through. Discard the rosemary.

4   Serve the turkey with the gravy accompanied by the Garlic Mashed Potatoes and Sautéed Sugar Snap Peas.

PER SERVING:

240 calories	45 g protein	5 g total carbohydrates	2 g fiber	3 g net carbohydrates

Turkey Marinara over Brown Rice

1 teaspoon olive oil

1 teaspoon minced garlic

12 ounces ground turkey

2 cups sugar-free marinara sauce

2 tablespoons chopped fresh basil

1/8 teaspoon dried oregano

Salt and fresh ground black pepper to taste

1 cup cooked brown rice

4 leaves fresh basil for garnish

1   Warm the oil in a 2-quart saucepan over medium heat. Add the garlic and sauté 30 seconds until fragrant; do not brown.

2   Add the turkey and cook, stirring occasionally until browned, 5 to 7 minutes.

3   Stir in the marinara sauce, basil, and oregano. Simmer uncovered until the sauce has thickened, 2 to 3 minutes. Season with salt and pepper.

4   Serve over the brown rice and garnish with the basil leaves.

PER SERVING:

322 calories	36 g protein	26 g total carbohydrates	2.5 g fiber	23.5 g net carbohydrates

Pesto-Grilled Chicken
with Sautéed Cauliflower

12 ounces uncooked skinless boneless chicken breasts

Pinch of red pepper flakes (optional)

½ teaspoon salt

Pinch of fresh ground black pepper

Lemon wedges for garnish

FOR THE PESTO:

1 cup basil leaves

⅓ cup olive oil

3 tablespoons low-sodium chicken stock or water

2 cloves garlic, peeled and halved

Salt and fresh ground pepper to taste

1   Preheat the oven to 375°F.

2   To make the pesto, place the basil, oil, stock or water, and garlic in a blender and puree until smooth. Season with salt and pepper.

3   Toss the chicken breasts with the pesto and refrigerate for at least 30 minutes or up to 2 hours.

4   Heat a nonstick grill pan over high heat. Scrape most of the pesto from the chicken and reserve. Grill the chicken for 3 minutes per side until lightly browned.

5   Transfer the chicken to a baking pan and spoon the reserved pesto over it.

6   Bake for 7 to 10 minutes until cooked through. Serve with Sautéed Cauliflower (page 115) and garnish with the lemon wedges.

SAUTÉED CAULIFLOWER

½ medium cauliflower, separated into florets

¾ cup low-sodium chicken stock

Salt and fresh ground black pepper to taste

1 teaspoon chopped fresh parsley

1   Heat a medium nonstick skillet over medium heat. Add the cauliflower and stock. Cook covered for 5 to 7 minutes.

2   Uncover the skillet and continue simmering over medium heat until all the stock has been absorbed and the cauliflower begins to brown. Season with salt and pepper, and sprinkle with parsley.

PER SERVING:

249 calories	44 g protein	12 g total carbohydrates	5.4 g fiber	6.6 g net carbohydrates

Spicy Catfish with Roasted Fennel and Spicy Sautéed String Beans

SERVES 2

1 large bulb fennel, trimmed and thinly sliced

2 teaspoons olive oil

Salt and fresh ground black pepper to taste

2 catfish fillets, about 6 ounces each

One 14-ounce can Italian peeled plum tomatoes with their juice

2 hot cherry peppers from a jar, sliced

1 tablespoon chopped fresh basil

1 tablespoon chopped fresh cilantro

1 recipe Spicy Sautéed String Beans (page 169)

1   Preheat the oven to 400°F.

2   Toss the fennel slices with the olive oil, and season with salt and pepper. Transfer the fennel to a 6 by 8-inch baking dish and roast 15 minutes, stirring occasionally for even browning.

3   Place the catfish on top of the fennel and season lightly with salt and pepper. Pour the tomatoes and peppers over the fish and sprinkle with the basil and cilantro.

4   Return the pan to the oven and bake for 15 minutes until the fish is cooked through. Serve with the Spicy Sautéed String Beans.

PER SERVING:

| 315 calories | 33 g protein | 23 g total carbohydrates | 7 g fiber | 16 g net carbohydrates |

Grilled Marinated Lamb and Vegetables with Mint Pesto and Seasoned Barley

8 ounces leg of lamb, trimmed and cubed

1 red bell pepper, cut into 1-inch pieces

1 large red onion, cut into 1-inch pieces

6 cherry tomatoes

½ cup low-sodium chicken stock

1 recipe Seasoned Barley (page 93)

FOR THE MINT PESTO:

½ cup chopped fresh mint

¼ cup olive oil

3 tablespoons low-sodium chicken stock

2 cloves garlic, peeled

½ teaspoon salt

Pinch of red pepper flakes

1   Blend the pesto ingredients in a blender until smooth.

2   Transfer the pesto to a large bowl. Toss in the lamb, pepper, onion, and tomatoes. Cover and refrigerate 2 hours or overnight.

3   Heat a grill pan over high heat. Transfer the lamb and vegetables to the pan, reserving the marinade. Grill 5 to 7 minutes until cooked to desired doneness.

4   Transfer the lamb and vegetables to a small saucepan. Add the reserved marinade and the chicken stock. Simmer over medium heat for 3 to 4 minutes. Serve over Seasoned Barley.

PER SERVING:

508 calories	21 g protein	37 g carbohydrates	5 g fiber	32 g net carbohydrates

Blue-Corn-Crusted Salmon with Spicy Sautéed Vegetable Medley

2 large handfuls blue corn chips

Two 4-ounce pieces salmon fillet, skin removed

4 tablespoons Dijon-style mustard

1   Preheat the oven to 375°F. Lightly coat a 6 by 8-inch baking dish with Pam.

2   Place the corn chips in a blender or food processor and grind to a coarse meal. Transfer the cornmeal to a plate.

3   Smear the salmon all over with the mustard and dredge in the cornmeal.

4   Transfer the salmon to the baking dish and bake for 15 minutes. Serve salmon over the Spicy Sautéed Vegetable Medley (page 119).

SPICY SAUTÉED VEGETABLE MEDLEY

1 teaspoon olive oil

1 clove garlic, crushed to a paste

¼ teaspoon red pepper flakes

1 cup low-sodium chicken stock

2 cups chopped escarole or kale

2 cups green beans, sliced into 1-inch pieces

2 cups broccoli florets

Salt and fresh ground black pepper to taste

1   Heat a 10- or 12-inch nonstick skillet over medium heat.

2   Add the oil, garlic, and red pepper flakes. Sizzle for 10 seconds until the garlic begins to turn golden. Pour in the stock and raise the heat to high.

3   Add the escarole or kale, green beans, and broccoli and bring to a boil. Reduce the heat to medium and simmer until nearly all the stock has cooked off. Season with salt and pepper. Serve immediately.

PER SERVING:

325 calories	30 g protein	19.1 g total carbohydrates	2.1 g fiber	17 g net carbohydrates

SETH WILLIAMS'S 5 SQUARES
MAKEOVER SUCCESS STORY

I HAVE HAD A WEIGHT PROBLEM my entire life. I was the only one in my family who did. I was a chubby kid and an overweight teen, and by high school I was downright fat. My friends called me "Tubs" and even though I tried to pretend that it was cool "livin' large," it wasn't. I couldn't meet girls who liked me as more than a friend or a shoulder to cry on. I wasn't fast enough to play sports.

By the time I was 25, I was morbidly obese and my parents forced me to see a nutritionist. The nutritionist put me on a special diet, but I didn't stick to it. In fact, I rebelled and ate more. Every time I went out with my friends, I would drink and eat junk food. The scale kept going up each time I visited the office and it became clear that the nutritionist was a waste of time. I had only gone to get my parents off my case. I had to get healthy for myself, not for my parents, but I didn't know how to go about it.

Finally, I met a girl who I really liked. She didn't seem to notice how big I was. Instead, she saw me underneath all those pounds. We became fast friends and one day we began talking about my weight issues. She told me she had been 75 pounds heavier and had lost the weight through a program called 5 squares. My friend said the food was really good and encouraged me by saying that it was easy to stick to the program.

I didn't start 5 squares for another four months. I thought about it carefully and one morning I just woke up and wanted to be different. I didn't want to struggle to walk anymore, or be embarrassed in public. I was a bit nervous at first, of course; there was a lot a food and I wanted to make sure I was doing the right thing. It never seemed like I was on a diet; the 5 squares staff actually encouraged me to eat by explaining that it wasn't the amount I was eating but the choices I was making. Monica Lynn showed me how to eat smaller meals throughout the day to keep my hunger down and my energy up. Surprisingly, I felt better almost immediately.

In fact, I felt so much better that I started walking. I took it slowly at first: I could barely walk a city block when I started. But by the third week, I could power-walk a mile and a half. I was on my way! My parents were so surprised. My father told me he never thought I would lose the weight. I cannot tell you how good it felt proving him wrong. After I lost 100 pounds, Monica Lynn helped me transition from her food to food that I could prepare myself. I had another 50 pounds to lose but she wanted to show me how easy it was for me to do it on my own. I was apprehensive, but with her encouragement, I stuck to it. I am now 30 years old and down to a healthy weight of 175 pounds.

I am in control of my health and my life. It is great to look in the mirror and be proud of what I see.

Spicy Roasted Pepper Soup with Chicken and Lime

SERVES 2

1 roasted red pepper from a jar

One 14-ounce can plum tomatoes with their juice

1 clove garlic, peeled

2½ cups low-sodium chicken stock

6 ounces uncooked skinless boneless chicken breast, sliced into ½-inch cubes

1 tablespoon fresh lime juice

Pinch of fresh ground black pepper

2 to 3 tablespoons chopped fresh cilantro

3 shakes of Tabasco or to taste

Salt to taste

1   Combine the red pepper, tomatoes with their juice, garlic, and ½ cup of the stock in a blender. Process until smooth.

2   Transfer the puree to a small saucepan and stir in the remaining stock. Bring to a boil over high heat.

3   Reduce the heat to medium and add the chicken. Simmer over medium heat for 10 minutes, stirring occasionally until the soup thickens slightly and the chicken is cooked through.

4   Stir in the lime juice, pepper, and cilantro. Season with Tabasco and salt. Serve hot.

PER SERVING:

| 179 calories | 23 g protein | 20 g total carbohydrates | 5 g fiber | 15 g net carbohydrates |

Chicken, Cauliflower, and Leek Soup

1 teaspoon olive oil

1 cup thinly sliced leek whites from 2 medium leeks

Pinch of salt

3 cups low-sodium chicken stock

2 cups roughly chopped cauliflower

3 ounces uncooked skinless boneless chicken breast, sliced into ½-inch pieces

2 teaspoons fresh lemon juice

1 teaspoon chopped fresh parsley

Fresh ground black pepper to taste

1   Heat the oil in a 1½- to 2-quart saucepan over medium heat. Add the leeks and a pinch of salt and sauté 5 minutes until they soften.

2   Add the stock and cauliflower. Raise the heat and bring to boil. Reduce the heat to low and simmer 10 minutes.

3   Add the chicken and simmer 6 to 8 minutes until cooked through. Stir in the lemon juice and parsley. Season with salt and pepper and serve.

PER SERVING:

| 132 calories | 14 g protein | 14 g total carbohydrates | 4 g fiber | 10 g net carbohydrates |

Chicken Salad Lettuce Wrap

6 ounces uncooked skinless boneless chicken breast, rinsed

1 tablespoon Nayonaise

1 tablespoon mustard

2 teaspoons distilled white vinegar

⅛ teaspoon Splenda (sugar-free sweetener)

2 tablespoons chopped celery

2 tablespoons chopped water chestnuts

8 seedless grapes, halved

¼ cup sliced almonds, lightly toasted (page 67)

Salt and fresh ground black pepper to taste

4 whole pieces Bibb lettuce, washed and dried

1   Bring 1 quart of lightly salted water to a boil in a medium covered saucepan. Add the chicken, reduce the heat to medium, and simmer covered for 8 to 10 minutes until cooked through.

2   Transfer the chicken to a plate and refrigerate for 1 hour.

3   In a large bowl, combine the Nayonaise, mustard, vinegar, and Splenda. Whisk until smooth.

4   Add the celery, water chestnuts, grapes, and almonds to the bowl.

5   Dice the cold chicken and transfer it to the bowl. Toss well and season with salt and fresh ground black pepper.

6   Mound the salad onto the lettuce leaves, roll up, and serve.

PER SERVING:

121 calories	23.25 g protein	5.08 g total carbohydrates	0.25 g fiber	4.83 g net carbohydrates

Escarole and White Bean Soup

Two 14-ounce cans low-sodium chicken stock

⅓ cup water

2 tablespoons finely chopped onion

2 cloves garlic, crushed to a paste

¼ teaspoon dried oregano

2 cups firmly packed chopped escarole

One 14-ounce can white beans, rinsed and drained

Salt and fresh ground black pepper to taste

1. In a 1½- to 2-quart saucepan combine the stock, water, onion, garlic, and oregano. Place the pan over high heat and bring to a boil.

2. Add the escarole and white beans. Reduce the heat to low when the soup resumes boiling. Simmer 10 to 15 minutes until the escarole is tender.

3. Season with salt and fresh ground black pepper. Serve immediately. You can freeze any leftovers.

PER SERVING:

107.7 calories	5.3 g protein	20.3 g total carbohydrates	5.8 g fiber	14.5 g net carbohydrates

Pesto Shrimp Cocktail

½ cup firmly packed basil leaves

¼ cup olive oil

2 tablespoons low-sodium chicken stock or water

1 clove garlic, peeled and halved

Small pinch of red pepper flakes (optional)

Salt and fresh ground black pepper to taste

8 ounces raw shrimp, peeled and deveined (preferably 16 to 20 count)

Lemon wedges for garnish

1   To make the pesto, puree the basil, oil, stock or water, garlic, and red pepper flakes in a blender until smooth. Season with salt and pepper.

2   Toss the shrimp with the pesto and refrigerate 30 minutes.

3   Preheat the oven to 375° F.

4   On a baking sheet, spread the shrimp with the marinade. Bake for 10 minutes until cooked through.

5   Serve shrimp hot or cold accompanied by lemon wedges.

PER SERVING:

379 calories	25 g protein	4 g total carbohydrates	1 g fiber	3 g net carbohydrates

Turkey Burger with Grilled Eggplant and Sautéed Zucchini

SERVES 2

12 ounces ground turkey

2½ teaspoons McCormick Grill Mates Roasted Garlic Montreal Chicken Seasoning blend

1 tablespoon chopped fresh cilantro

2 large slices eggplant, about ½ inch thick

1 tablespoon sugar-free balsamic vinegar

Pinch of dried oregano

Salt and fresh ground black pepper to taste

1 small onion, thinly sliced, about ½ cup

1 medium zucchini, thinly sliced, about 1½ cups

1   Preheat the oven to 375°F.

2   Toss the turkey with the roasted garlic seasoning and cilantro. Form into 2 patties.

3   Heat a nonstick grill pan over medium heat. Lightly spray with Pam and grill burgers 2 minutes per side. Transfer the burgers to a baking sheet and bake them in the oven for 7 to 8 minutes until cooked through.

4   Return the grill pan to the heat. In a small bowl toss the eggplant slices with the balsamic vinegar and oregano. Season with salt and pepper. Grill for 2 minutes per side until tender.

5   Lightly coat an 8- to 10-inch nonstick skillet with Pam and place over high heat. Add the onion and zucchini. Season with a pinch of salt and pepper and sauté 5 minutes, stirring occasionally, until lightly browned.

6   Serve the burgers topped with eggplant and accompanied by the sautéed vegetables.

PER SERVING:

226 calories	40 g protein	8 g total carbohydrates	4 g fiber	4 g net carbohydrates

Chicken, Barley, and Vegetable Soup

SERVES 2

3 cups low-sodium chicken stock

2 tablespoons barley

1 cup chopped mixed vegetables, such as zucchini, string beans, carrots

6 ounces uncooked skinless boneless chicken breast, sliced into ½-inch pieces

1 teaspoon chopped fresh dill

Salt and fresh ground black pepper to taste

1 teaspoon chopped fresh parsley

1   Combine the stock and barley in a medium saucepan. Place the pan over high heat and bring to a boil. Reduce the heat to low, cover, and simmer for 30 minutes or until the barley is tender.

2   Add the vegetables, chicken, and dill and simmer 10 to 15 minutes until the vegetables are tender and the chicken is cooked through.

3   Season the soup with salt and pepper. Stir in the parsley and serve.

PER SERVING:

158 calories	25 g protein	17 g total carbohydrates	5 g fiber	12 g net carbohydrates

Barbecued Salmon with Braised Cabbage

SERVES 2

Two 4-ounce salmon fillets

2 tablespoons sugar- and calorie-free barbecue sauce

1 teaspoon olive oil

3 cups thinly sliced red cabbage

Pinch of salt

½ cup low-sodium chicken stock

1 tablespoon distilled white vinegar

1 tablespoon chopped fresh dill

Fresh ground black pepper to taste

1   Toss the salmon with the barbecue sauce and refrigerate 1 hour or overnight.

2   Preheat the oven to 400°F.

3   Place the salmon with its marinade in a small nonstick baking pan. Bake 12 to 14 minutes until the desired doneness is reached.

4   Meanwhile, in an 8- or 10-inch nonstick sauté pan over medium heat, add the oil, cabbage, and a pinch of salt. Sauté 2 minutes, stirring frequently, until the cabbage begins to soften.

5   Add the chicken stock and vinegar to the pan and simmer covered for 10 minutes until the cabbage is tender. Stir in the dill and season with salt and pepper.

6   Serve the salmon with the braised cabbage on the side.

PER SERVING:

252 calories	24 g protein	5 g total carbohydrates	5 g fiber	0 g net carbohydrates

Julienned Turkey Chef Salad

4 romaine leaves

4 cups prewashed mesclun greens

4 tablespoons sugar-free Thousand Island dressing, plus additional to taste

3 ounces Canadian bacon, julienned, about ¾ cup

3 ounces fresh roasted turkey breast, julienned, about ¾ cup

1 hard-boiled egg, quartered

4 cherry tomatoes, halved

½ medium cucumber, cut into 6 to 8 slices

1   Divide the romaine leaves between two plates.

2   Toss the mesclun with the 4 tablespoons dressing and mound it over the romaine. Arrange the bacon and turkey over the greens. Garnish with the egg, tomatoes, and cucumbers. Serve the salads with additional dressing on the side.

PER SERVING:

243 calories	30 g protein	8 g total carbohydrates	3 g fiber	5 g net carbohydrates

Double-Mustard Chicken
and Arugula Salad

SERVES 2

6 ounces uncooked skinless boneless chicken breast

½ teaspoon salt

⅛ teaspoon fresh ground black pepper

2 tablespoons spicy brown mustard or grainy Dijon mustard

3 tablespoons calorie- and sugar-free honey-Dijon dressing

1 teaspoon olive oil

3 cups lightly packed arugula, washed and dried

2 tablespoons chopped walnuts (optional)

1   Season the chicken with the salt and pepper. Place the chicken in a bowl, adding the spicy brown or grainy Dijon mustard and 1 tablespoon of the honey-Dijon dressing. Coat the chicken with the mustard and dressing and refrigerate for 30 minutes or overnight.

2   Preheat the oven to 375°F.

3   Heat an 8-inch ovenproof nonstick skillet over medium heat until hot. Add the oil and chicken. Cook for 3 minutes on one side. Turn the chicken over and cook 1 minute more. Transfer the skillet to the oven for 8 to 10 minutes until the chicken is cooked through.

4   Transfer the chicken to a plate and cool until warm. Slice into thin strips.

5   In a large mixing bowl toss the arugula with the remaining 2 tablespoons honey-Dijon dressing.

6   Mound the arugula onto two plates and top with the sliced chicken. If desired, sprinkle the salads with walnuts before serving.

PER SERVING:

124 calories	20.5 g protein	1.75 g total carbohydrates	0.75 g fiber	1 g net carbohydrate

Chopped Chicken Salad with Creamy Lemon-Dill Vinaigrette

SERVES 2

3 cups lightly salted water

8 ounces uncooked skinless boneless chicken breast

2 tablespoons Nayonaise

1 tablespoon fresh lemon juice

1 tablespoon chopped fresh dill

⅛ teaspoon Splenda (sugar-free sweetener)

1 yellow bell pepper, cored and diced

1 small cucumber, peeled and diced

1 small carrot, peeled and coarsely grated

1 heart of romaine, chopped

2 tablespoons chopped walnuts

1 tablespoon raisins

Salt and fresh ground black pepper to taste

1   Bring 3 cups lightly salted water to a boil in a 1½- to 2-quart saucepan. Add the chicken and cover the pan. Simmer over medium heat for 7 to 8 minutes until cooked through. Drain the chicken in a sieve and cool under cold running water. Drain well and chop into small pieces.

2   In a mixing bowl whisk the Nayonaise, lemon juice, dill, and Splenda until smooth.

3   Add the chicken, bell pepper, cucumber, carrot, romaine, walnuts, and raisins. Toss well and season with salt and pepper. Refrigerate, and serve cold.

PER SERVING:

266 calories	30.4 g protein	18 g total carbohydrates	3.26 g fiber	14.74 g net carbohydrates

Seafood Salad

SERVES 2

4 ounces small shrimp, peeled and deveined, about ½ cup

4 ounces tiny bay scallops, about ½ cup

1 tablespoon distilled white vinegar

2 tablespoons fresh lemon juice

½ teaspoon salt

⅛ teaspoon fresh ground pepper

1 tablespoon chopped fresh parsley

1 tablespoon chopped fresh dill

1 teaspoon olive oil

½ cup cucumber, peeled, seeded, and diced

4 cherry tomatoes, quartered

1 head Boston or Bibb lettuce separated into 4 lettuce cups

Lemon wedges for garnish

1   Steam the shrimp and scallops over ½ inch of boiling water in a covered pan for 2 to 3 minutes until cooked through. Drain the seafood in a sieve and cool under cold running water. Drain well.

2   Place the vinegar, lemon juice, salt, pepper, parsley, dill, olive oil, cucumber, and tomatoes in a bowl and toss to combine. Mix in the seafood and chill for at least 15 minutes to allow the flavors to marry.

3   Serve the salad in lettuce cups, garnished with lemon wedges.

PER SERVING:

154 calories	21 g protein	8.35 g total carbohydrates	0.13 g fiber	8.22 g net carbohydrates

Pulled Chicken Salad with Peppers, Eggplant, and Spelt Croutons

SERVES 2

8 ounces uncooked skinless boneless chicken breast

2 tablespoons calorie- and sugar-free sun-dried tomato dressing

1 teaspoon dried basil

Salt and fresh ground black pepper to taste

1 medium eggplant, trimmed and cubed, about 2 cups

2 tablespoons sugar-free balsamic vinegar

2 teaspoons olive oil

1 roasted red pepper from a jar, thinly sliced

2 teaspoons capers

2 tablespoons chopped fresh basil

½ teaspoon dried oregano

1 slice spelt bread, cut into ½-inch cubes

2 cups prewashed mesclun greens

4 cherry tomatoes, halved

1 Preheat the oven to 400°F.

2 Steam the chicken over ½ inch of boiling water in a covered pan for 10 to 12 minutes until cooked through. Transfer to a plate to cool. Shred the chicken into long strips and toss with the sun-dried tomato dressing and basil. Season with salt and pepper and set aside.

3 Toss the eggplant with ½ teaspoon salt, the balsamic vinegar, and 1 teaspoon of the oil. Spread the eggplant on a 6 by 8-inch baking dish and roast for 15 minutes until tender.

4 Transfer the eggplant to a bowl. Add the roasted pepper, capers, fresh basil, and dried oregano. Toss to combine and season with salt and pepper.

5   Spread the bread on a cookie sheet and toss with the remaining teaspoon of olive oil. Toast in the oven for 10 minutes, stirring halfway for even browning. Transfer the croutons to a plate to cool and crisp.

6   Divide the mesclun between two plates. Top each with a mound of roasted eggplant. Arrange the chicken strips around the eggplant. Scatter the croutons over all and garnish with cherry tomatoes.

PER SERVING:

200 calories	28.05 g protein	12.9 g total carbohydrates	4 g fiber	8.9 g net carbohydrates

Turkey Burger with Sautéed Mushrooms

SERVES 2

12 ounces ground turkey

2½ teaspoons McCormick Grill Mates Roasted Garlic Montreal Chicken Seasoning blend

1 teaspoon fresh thyme

1 tablespoon chopped fresh cilantro

1 teaspoon olive oil

1 teaspoon minced garlic

6 ounces button mushrooms, halved, about 2 cups

1 tablespoon low-sodium chicken stock

1 teaspoon chopped fresh parsley

1   Preheat the oven to 375°F.

2   Toss the turkey with the roasted garlic seasoning, thyme, and cilantro. Form into 2 patties.

3   Heat a nonstick grill pan over medium heat. Lightly spray it with Pam and grill the burgers 2 minutes per side. Transfer the burgers to a baking sheet and bake them in the oven for 7 to 8 minutes until cooked through.

4   Place a small nonstick skillet over medium heat. Add the oil and garlic and sauté for 30 seconds; do not brown.

5   Add the mushrooms and sauté 2 to 3 minutes, stirring occasionally, until lightly browned.

6   Add the chicken stock and simmer until nearly dry. Season with salt and pepper and toss with the parsley.

7   Serve the burgers with the mushrooms on the side.

PER SERVING:

| 220 calories | 33.7 g protein | 2 g total carbohydrates | 1 g fiber | 1 g net carbohydrates |

Pulled Turkey Salad with Arugula, Garbanzos, and Red Onion

SERVES 2

8 ounces fresh turkey cutlets

Salt and fresh ground black pepper to taste

3 to 4 tablespoons sugar- and calorie-free balsamic dressing

1 bunch arugula, trimmed and washed, about 4 cups

1 small red onion, thinly sliced, about ⅓ cup

½ cup canned garbanzo beans, rinsed and drained

3 cherry tomatoes, halved

1 Preheat the oven to 375°F.

2 Spray a 12-inch square of aluminum foil with Pam. Place the turkey on the foil and season lightly with salt and pepper. Crimp the foil to form a neat package. Bake 20 to 25 minutes until cooked through. Transfer the turkey to a plate to cool.

3 Pull the turkey into long shreds and toss with 1 tablespoon of the balsamic dressing.

4 Toss the arugula and red onion with the remaining dressing to taste.

5 Mound the arugula onto two plates and top with the turkey. Sprinkle with the garbanzos and garnish with the cherry tomatoes.

PER SERVING:

194 calories	31 g protein	13.5 g total carbohydrates	4 g fiber	9.5 g net carbohydrates

Chicken and Roasted Pepper Salad

6 ounces uncooked skinless boneless chicken breast, butterflied

Salt and fresh ground black pepper to taste

1 roasted red pepper from a jar, cut into ½-inch strips

2 cloves garlic, crushed

½ teaspoon dried oregano

¼ teaspoon red pepper flakes

2 teaspoons capers, drained

1 teaspoon olive oil

4 cups prewashed mesclun greens

Sugar-free dressing of your choice to taste

4 cherry tomatoes, halved

1 small carrot, peeled and cut into curls with a vegetable peeler

1 Preheat the oven to 375°F. Lightly spray a 6 by 8-inch baking dish with Pam.

2 On a clean work surface, season the chicken with salt and pepper.

3 In a small bowl toss the pepper strips with the garlic, oregano, red pepper flakes, capers, and olive oil.

4 Lay the pepper strips over the chicken and roll up the chicken to encompass the filling. Spray lightly with Pam.

5 Place the chicken in the baking dish, seam side down, and bake 25 minutes or until cooked through.

6 Transfer the chicken to a clean cutting surface and cool.

7 Toss the mesclun greens with the dressing to taste and mound onto two plates. Slice the chicken and place it on top of the greens. Serve garnished with tomatoes and carrot curls.

PER SERVING:

129.8 calories	20.2 g protein	8 g total carbohydrates	1.35 g fiber	6.65 g net carbohydrates

Three-Bean Salad

One 14-ounce can three-bean mix, drained and rinsed

2 tablespoons sugar-free balsamic dressing

1 tablespoon finely chopped red onion

2 tablespoons chopped fresh basil

1 teaspoon lemon juice

1 teaspoon olive oil

½ teaspoon salt

Pinch of fresh ground black pepper

Combine all the ingredients in a bowl and mix well. Serve as prepared or with 8 to 10 of your favorite corn tortilla chips.

PER SERVING:

184 calories	7 g protein	15.3 g total carbohydrates	8 g fiber	7.3 g net carbohydrates

Bean Salad with Canadian Bacon and Roasted Peppers

SERVES 2

4 ounces Canadian bacon

One 14-ounce can three-bean mix, drained and rinsed

1 roasted red pepper from a jar, diced

1 tablespoon thinly sliced red onion

2 tablespoons chopped fresh parsley

1 tablespoon distilled white vinegar

2 shakes of Tabasco or to taste

1 teaspoon olive oil

Salt to taste

Sliced cucumber for garnish

1 tomato, cut into wedges

1   Heat a grill pan over medium heat until hot. Grill bacon 2 minutes per side. Transfer to a cutting surface and dice.

2   Combine the bacon, beans, diced pepper, and onion in a large bowl. Add the parsley, vinegar, Tabasco, and oil. Toss well and season with salt.

3   Serve the salad garnished with sliced cucumbers and the tomato wedges.

PER SERVING:

283.8 calories	19.5 g protein	16.8 g total carbohydrates	10 g fiber	6.8 g net carbohydrates

Chicken Sautéed with Peppers, Eggplant, and Mushrooms

SERVES 2

6 ounces uncooked skinless boneless chicken breast, sliced into
    ½-inch strips

Juice and zest of ½ lemon

1 clove garlic, crushed to a paste

2 teaspoons chopped fresh rosemary

½ teaspoon salt

Pinch of fresh ground black pepper

2 teaspoons canola oil

1 cup low-sodium chicken stock

2 teaspoons wheat-free tamari soy sauce

2 cups diced eggplant

2 cups thinly sliced mushrooms

1 red bell pepper, cored and thinly sliced

1 tablespoon chopped fresh parsley for garnish

1   Toss the chicken strips with the lemon juice, zest, garlic, and rosemary. Season with ½ teaspoon salt and a pinch of black pepper.

2   Heat a 10- or 12-inch nonstick skillet over medium heat. Add the oil and chicken and raise the heat to high. Sear the chicken 2 to 3 minutes until golden brown all over. Transfer the chicken to a plate.

3   Pour the stock and tamari into the skillet and bring to a boil. Add the eggplant, mushrooms, and pepper. Reduce the heat to medium and simmer 5 to 7 minutes until the vegetables are tender.

4   Return the chicken and any juices to the pan and simmer 1 minute. Season with salt and pepper, sprinkle with parsley, and serve.

PER SERVING:

169 calories	24 g protein	9.7 g total carbohydrates	4.55 g fiber	5.15 g net carbohydrates

Balsamic-Glazed Tuna with Sweet and Sour Cucumbers

SERVES 2

Two 6-ounce tuna steaks, about ¾ inch thick

1¼ teaspoons cracked black pepper

¼ teaspoon salt

¼ cup low-sodium chicken stock

1 tablespoon sugar-free balsamic vinegar

⅛ teaspoon Splenda (sugar-free sweetener)

1 tablespoon wheat-free tamari soy sauce

½ teaspoon cornstarch

2 scallions, thinly sliced, about ¼ cup

1 recipe Sweet and Sour Cucumbers (page 80)

1 Lightly spray a nonstick grill pan with Pam and place over medium-high heat.

2 Sprinkle the steaks on both sides with the pepper and salt.

3 Grill the tuna for 3 minutes on each side until medium-rare or to desired doneness. Remove the pan from the heat.

4 Combine the stock, vinegar, Splenda, tamari, and cornstarch in a small pan. Bring to a boil over medium heat. Reduce the heat to low and cook for 1 minute, stirring constantly.

5 Spoon the glaze over the fish and garnish with sliced scallions. Serve with Sweet and Sour Cucumbers.

PER SERVING:

264 calories	48 g protein	10 g total carbohydrates	4 g fiber	6 g net carbohydrates

ANTOINETTE CALDERON'S 5 SQUARES MAKEOVER SUCCESS STORY

WHEN OPPORTUNITY KNOCKS, YOU SHOULD ANSWER. I feel like one of the luckiest people in the world right now, especially due to the help of 5 squares. Someone very close to me introduced me to 5 squares and offered me an opportunity. I was at a point in my life where nothing was going right, I was in a funk, work stank, and I was filled to the brim with negativity. I shot up to 243 pounds and, being a vertically challenged woman of five two, I knew my situation would not change easily. During my first week on 5 squares, I called every five minutes to ask a question. I was pessimistic, and did not want to eat all the food we were required to each day. As delicious as it was, I thought I was eating too much. Still, I forged ahead and promised myself I would stick with it for at least a week.

At the end of the week, the scale revealed that I'd lost 8 pounds and I *screamed* for joy. I was hooked on 5 squares and on the motivation to feel better. I am now down 64 pounds with a body that has replaced fat mass with a thrilling amount of muscle mass. I still have more weight to go, and I would like to lose another 50 pounds, so I am willfully working toward it. But my head is clear and my confidence has sky-rocketed—5 squares made me realize that there is a healthy way to lose weight and live a better life.

SQUARE 5

Stuffed Tomatoes with Garlic Sautéed Broccoli

12 ounces ground turkey

1 large egg, lightly beaten

2 teaspoons finely chopped fresh parsley

1 teaspoon dried oregano

2 tablespoons quick oats

4 tablespoons sugar-free marinara sauce

1 teaspoon olive oil

2 tablespoons finely chopped onion

2 cloves garlic, crushed to a paste

Pinch of salt

Fresh ground black pepper to taste

1 large beefsteak tomato, sliced in half, pulp and seeds discarded

1   Preheat the oven to 375°F.

2   In a large bowl combine the turkey, egg, parsley, oregano, oats, and marinara sauce.

3   Warm the oil in a small sauté pan over medium heat. Add the onion, garlic, and a pinch of salt. Sauté for 2 to 3 minutes until lightly browned. Transfer the onion and garlic to the bowl with the turkey and mix well. Season with salt and pepper.

4   Mound the turkey mixture into the tomato halves. Place the stuffed tomatoes in a pie plate or small baking dish lightly coated with nonstick cooking spray and bake for 25 minutes until cooked through. Serve with Garlic Sautéed Broccoli (page 149).

Note: For variety, try adding 1 tablespoon chopped walnuts and 1 tablespoon chopped raisins to the stuffing.

GARLIC SAUTÉED BROCCOLI

1 teaspoon olive oil

1 clove garlic, crushed to a paste

1 pinch of red pepper flakes

2 cups small broccoli florets

¼ cup low-sodium chicken stock

Salt to taste

1   Warm the oil in a medium nonstick skillet over medium heat. Add the garlic and red pepper flakes, sizzle 10 seconds.

2   Add the broccoli and stock. Sauté 5 to 7 minutes until the broccoli is tender and bright green.

3   Season with salt and serve.

PER SERVING:

325 calories	41.3 g protein	12.4 g total carbohydrates	4.4 g fiber	8 g net carbohydrates

Filet Mignon with Garlic Mashed Potatoes and Sautéed Summer Squash

SERVES 2

1 teaspoon olive oil

8 ounces filet mignon

½ teaspoon salt

Fresh ground black pepper to taste

1   Preheat the oven to 400°F.

2   Place a small ovenproof nonstick skillet over high heat until very hot.

3   Add the oil and meat and sear all over for 3 to 4 minutes until well browned.

4   Transfer the skillet to the oven and roast 3 to 4 minutes for medium-rare.

5   Transfer the meat to a cutting surface and season all over with the salt and pepper. Cover the meat loosely with foil and let rest 4 to 5 minutes before slicing. Serve with the Garlic Mashed Potatoes and Sautéed Summer Squash (page 151).

GARLIC MASHED POTATOES

1 small Idaho potato, about 8 ounces, peeled and quartered

2 cloves garlic, peeled and left whole

2 cups cold water

¼ cup low-sodium chicken stock

Salt and fresh ground black pepper to taste

2 teaspoons chopped fresh parsley

1   Place the potato, garlic, and cold water in a 1- to 2-quart saucepan. Bring to a boil over high heat. Reduce the heat to low and simmer 12 to 15 minutes until the potato pierces easily with a fork. Remove from the heat.

2   Drain the potato and garlic and return them to the warm pan. Add the stock and mash until smooth. Season with salt and pepper. Stir in the parsley and serve.

SAUTÉED SUMMER SQUASH

1 teaspoon olive oil

1 clove garlic, crushed to a paste

1 medium yellow summer squash, thinly sliced, about 2 cups

2 tablespoons low-sodium chicken stock or water

Salt and fresh ground black pepper to taste

1   Heat a medium nonstick skillet over medium heat. Sizzle the garlic in the oil for 10 seconds. Add the squash and stock or water.

2   Cook over medium heat 5 minutes, stirring occasionally, until tender. Season with salt and pepper and serve.

PER SERVING:

| 210 calories | 27.5 g protein | 12.9 g total carbohydrates | 3.4 g fiber | 9.5 g net carbohydrates |

Chicken Quesadilla with Fresh Tomato Salsa and White Bean and Artichoke Dip

SERVES 2

12 ounces uncooked skinless boneless chicken breast

Salt and fresh ground black pepper to taste

2 fresh corn tortillas

1 cup shredded heart of romaine

2 tablespoons shredded soy cheese (optional)

1 recipe Fresh Tomato Salsa (page 39)

1   Steam the chicken in a covered pan over ½ inch of boiling water for 10 to 12 minutes until cooked through. Transfer the chicken to a plate to cool.

2   Pull the chicken into strips and toss with the salsa. Season with salt and pepper.

3   Heat a griddle over medium heat until hot. Toast the tortillas for 1 to 2 minutes per side until crisp.

4   Place a toasted tortilla on each of two plates. Top with the chicken-salsa mix. Mound the shredded lettuce and shredded soy cheese over the chicken. Serve the White Bean and Artichoke Dip (page 153) on the side.

WHITE BEAN AND ARTICHOKE DIP

One 14-ounce can Great Northern beans

2 cloves garlic, crushed to a paste

⅛ teaspoon red pepper flakes

¼ teaspoon dried oregano

1 teaspoon distilled white vinegar

1 tablespoon chopped fresh cilantro

2 to 3 tablespoons water

2 canned artichoke hearts, sliced

Salt to taste

1   In a 1- to 2-quart saucepan combine the beans with their juice, garlic, red pepper flakes, oregano, and vinegar. Simmer over medium heat for 2 to 3 minutes until heated through.

2   Stir in the cilantro, water, and artichokes. Simmer 2 minutes then mash with the back of a spoon. Season with salt and serve.

PER SERVING:

288 calories	52 g protein	18 g total carbohydrates	9.5 g fiber	8.5 g net carbohydrates

Garlic and Herb-Crusted Pork with Roasted Butternut Squash and Sautéed Broccoli Rabe

SERVES 2

1 teaspoon dried oregano

1 teaspoon dried basil

1 teaspoon dried thyme

½ teaspoon salt

¼ teaspoon fresh ground black pepper

8 ounces pork tenderloin

3 cloves garlic, crushed

1 teaspoon olive oil

1   Preheat the oven to 375°F. Lightly spray a 6 by 8-inch baking dish with Pam.

2   Combine the oregano, basil, thyme, ¼ teaspoon of the salt, and ⅛ teaspoon of the black pepper on a plate and set it aside.

3   Season the pork with the remaining salt and pepper. Rub with the garlic and oil. Roll the pork in the reserved herb mixture to coat.

4   Transfer the pork to the prepared baking dish and bake 25 to 30 minutes until cooked through to an internal temperature of 140°F. Transfer the pork to a cutting surface. Cover loosely with foil and rest for 5 minutes before slicing. Serve with Roasted Butternut Squash and Sautéed Broccoli Rabe (page 155).

ROASTED BUTTERNUT SQUASH

⅓ medium butternut squash, peeled and cut into ½-inch cubes, about 1 cup

1 teaspoon olive oil

¼ teaspoon salt

Pinch of fresh ground black pepper

¼ teaspoon dried basil

1. Preheat the oven to 375°F. Lightly spray a pie plate or small baking dish with Pam.

2. Toss the squash with the oil, salt, pepper, and basil. Transfer to the baking dish and roast 30 minutes until tender and golden brown.

SAUTÉED BROCCOLI RABE

2 quarts water

1 bunch broccoli rabe, tough stems discarded, roughly chopped

1 teaspoon olive oil

⅛ teaspoon red pepper flakes

1 clove garlic, thinly sliced

½ cup low-sodium chicken stock

Salt to taste

1. Bring the water to a boil in a 4- to 6-quart pot. Add the broccoli rabe and cook 2 to 3 minutes until it begins to soften. Drain.

2. Heat an 8- to 10-inch skillet over medium heat. Add the oil, red pepper flakes, and garlic. Sizzle for 30 seconds, then add the broccoli rabe and chicken stock. Cover the pan and cook over medium heat for 3 to 4 minutes until the broccoli rabe is tender and most of the stock has been absorbed. Season with salt and serve.

PER SERVING:

220 calories	15.2 g protein	11.4 g total carbohydrates	4 g fiber	7.4 g net carbohydrates

Chilean Sea Bass with Mint and Lemon Zest and Roasted Zucchini, Shallots, and Asparagus

SERVES 2

2 pieces Chilean sea bass, about 6 ounces each

1 clove garlic, crushed to a paste

½ teaspoon salt

⅛ teaspoon fresh ground black pepper

1 tablespoon low-sodium chicken stock

Juice and zest of 1 small lemon

1 teaspoon McCormick Lemon & Pepper Seasoning Salt

1 tablespoon chopped fresh mint

1   Preheat the oven to 375°F. Lightly spray a 6 by 8-inch baking dish with Pam.

2   Rub the fish all over with garlic and season with the salt and pepper. Transfer to the baking dish.

3   Pour in the stock and lemon juice. Sprinkle the fish with the lemon pepper seasoning, lemon zest, and mint.

4   Bake for 20 minutes until cooked through.

5   Serve with Roasted Zucchini, Shallots, and Asparagus (page 157).

ROASTED ZUCCHINI, SHALLOTS, AND ASPARAGUS

1 cup sliced zucchini, cut into ½-inch thick bite-size pieces

½ cup thinly sliced shallots

4 spears asparagus, sliced into 1-inch pieces

1 teaspoon olive oil

½ teaspoon salt

¼ teaspoon fresh ground black pepper

1 Preheat the oven to 375°F. Spray a small baking dish lightly with Pam.

2 Toss the zucchini, shallots, and asparagus with the oil, salt, and pepper. Transfer to the baking dish and roast 20 minutes until golden brown. Stir once or twice for even browning.

PER SERVING:

240 calories	36 g protein	13 g total carbohydrates	1.6 g fiber	11.4 g net carbohydrates

Sole à la Française with Sautéed Spinach

1 cup low-sodium chicken stock

½ lemon, thinly sliced

1 tablespoon chopped fresh dill

2 teaspoons cornstarch dissolved in 1 tablespoon cold water

Salt and fresh ground black pepper to taste

2 sole fillets, about 6 ounces each

½ cup egg whites

1 tablespoon chopped fresh parsley

Lemon wedges for garnish

1 recipe Sautéed Spinach (page 105)

1   To make the sauce, combine the stock, lemon slices, and dill in a small saucepan and place over high heat. When the stock boils, reduce the heat to low and simmer gently for 5 minutes.

2   Remove the lemon slices. Stir in the cornstarch mixture and cook 1 minute until the sauce thickens. Season with salt and pepper.

3   Place the fish on a plate and season with salt and pepper. Pour the egg whites into a shallow bowl or a pie plate.

4   Spray a large nonstick skillet with Pam and place over medium heat.

5   Dip the fish into the egg whites, add them to the skillet, and cook 3 minutes on each side until golden brown. Pour in the sauce, sprinkle with the parsley, and simmer over medium heat 1 minute. Serve hot with lemon wedges and with Sautéed Spinach.

PER SERVING:

197 calories	38 g protein	6 g total carbohydrates	3 g fiber	3 g net carbohydrates

Horseradish-and-Oat-Crusted Pork Loin with Rosemary Gravy and Steamed Asparagus

SERVES 2

4 tablespoons uncooked oatmeal (we use quick oats)

¼ teaspoon dried basil

¼ teaspoon dried thyme

½ teaspoon salt

¼ teaspoon fresh ground black pepper

8 ounces boneless pork loin, trimmed

2 cloves garlic, crushed to a paste

½ teaspoon dried oregano

1 teaspoon olive oil

2 tablespoons prepared horseradish

1 recipe Rosemary Gravy (page 112)

1 recipe Steamed Asparagus (page 94)

1   Preheat the oven to 375°F. Lightly spray a 6 by 8-inch baking dish with Pam.

2   Combine the oats, basil, thyme, ¼ teaspoon of the salt, and ⅛ teaspoon of the black pepper in a blender and grind to a meal. Transfer to a plate.

3   Season the pork with the remaining salt and pepper. Rub the pork with garlic, oregano, and oil. Smear all over with horseradish, then dredge in the oatmeal mixture.

4   Transfer the pork to the prepared baking dish and bake 25 to 30 minutes until cooked through to an internal temperature of 140°F. Serve with warm Rosemary Gravy and Steamed Asparagus.

PER SERVING:

256 calories	24.32 g protein	12.8 g total carbohydrates	3 g fiber	9.8 g net carbohydrates

Orange Roughy Marinara with Caponata

SERVES 2

2 orange roughy fillets, about 6 ounces each

1 clove garlic, crushed to a paste

½ teaspoon salt

¼ teaspoon fresh ground black pepper

2 tablespoons low-sodium chicken stock

1 tablespoon chopped fresh basil

1 cup sugar-free marinara sauce

1 Preheat the oven to 375°F. Lightly spray a 6 by 8-inch baking dish with Pam.

2 Rub the fillets with the garlic, salt, and pepper. Transfer the fish to the baking dish.

3 Pour in the stock. Scatter the basil over the fish and spread with the marinara sauce.

4 Bake 15 to 20 minutes or until cooked through. Serve with Caponata (below).

CAPONATA

SERVES 2–4

2 cups diced eggplant

2 cloves garlic, crushed to a paste

1 cup low-sodium chicken stock

⅛ teaspoon red pepper flakes

3 canned plum tomatoes, with their juice (3 tablespoons), roughly chopped

1 roasted red pepper from a jar, diced

2 tablespoons chopped fresh basil

1 teaspoon chopped fresh parsley

Salt to taste

1 Combine the eggplant, garlic, and chicken stock in a saucepan. Bring to a simmer over medium heat and cook until almost all the stock has been absorbed and the eggplant is tender, approximately 7 to 10 minutes.

2 Add the red pepper flakes, tomatoes with their juice, and diced pepper. Return to a simmer. Add the basil and parsley. Simmer for 2 minutes. Season with salt and serve.

PER SERVING:

| 199 calories | 31 g protein | 17.5 g total carbohydrates | 5.5 g fiber | 12 g net carbohydrates |

Orange Roughy Provençal with Rosemary-Roasted Potatoes

2 orange roughy fillets, 6 ounces each

1 clove garlic, crushed to a paste

Salt and fresh ground black pepper to taste

2 canned plum tomatoes with 4 tablespoons of their juice

2 tablespoons low-sodium chicken stock

2 bottled artichoke hearts, halved

1 teaspoon capers

1 tablespoon chopped fresh basil

1 recipe Rosemary-Roasted Potatoes (page 91)

1   Preheat the oven to 375°F. Lightly spray a 6 by 8-inch baking dish with Pam.

2   Place the fillets in the baking dish. Rub with the garlic and lightly sprinkle with salt and pepper.

3   Lightly crush the tomatoes with the back of a spoon and place them on top of the fish. Spoon their juice and the stock over them.

4   Place 2 artichoke halves on each fillet and sprinkle them with capers and basil.

5   Bake 15 to 20 minutes until cooked through. Serve with Rosemary-Roasted Potatoes.

PER SERVING:

223.5 calories	30.5 g protein	14.85 g total carbohydrates	6.5 g fiber	8.35 g net carbohydrates

Turkey Vegetable Stir-Fry with Rice Noodles

SERVES 2

1 teaspoon oil

1 teaspoon finely chopped ginger

2 teaspoons finely chopped garlic

Pinch of red pepper flakes (optional)

1 teaspoon sesame seeds (optional)

1½ cups broccoli florets

½ cup sliced celery

½ cup thinly sliced onion

2 tablespoons low-sodium chicken stock

12 ounces turkey cutlets, sliced into thin strips

2 tablespoons wheat-free tamari sauce or to taste

1 ounce wide rice noodles, cooked according to directions on package (see Note below)

2 tablespoons chopped fresh cilantro

1   Heat a wok or wide nonstick skillet over high heat. Add the oil, ginger, garlic, red pepper flakes, if using, and sesame seeds, if using, and sizzle for 10 to 15 seconds.

2   Add the broccoli, celery, onion, and chicken stock. Stir-fry 3 to 4 minutes until the vegetables begin to soften.

3   Add the turkey and stir-fry 3 to 4 minutes until cooked through. Season with tamari and stir in the cooked noodles. Stir in the cilantro and serve.

Note: Wide rice noodles can be found in Asian supermarkets or the ethnic section of most large supermarkets.

PER SERVING:

352 calories	46 g protein	35.2 g total carbohydrates	5 g fiber	30.2 g net carbohydrates

Stuffed Sole with Asparagus and Mushrooms and Sautéed Sliced Potato and Onion

SERVES 2

8 slender spears asparagus, trimmed

1 teaspoon olive oil

2 cloves garlic, crushed to a paste

1 cup thinly sliced mushrooms

¾ cup low-sodium chicken stock

2 sole fillets, about 6 ounces each

½ teaspoon salt

¼ teaspoon fresh ground black pepper

1 tablespoon fresh lemon juice

Paprika to taste

2 teaspoons chopped fresh parsley

1   Preheat the oven to 375°F. Lightly spray a 6 by 8-inch baking dish with Pam.

2   Steam the asparagus over a ½ inch of boiling water in a covered pan for 2 to 3 minutes until bright green and tender.

3   In a skillet over medium heat sauté the oil and garlic 30 seconds until golden. Add the mushrooms and sauté, stirring occasionally, for 2 minutes until softened. Add ½ cup of the stock and asparagus and cook 3 to 5 minutes or until vegetables are tender. Transfer the vegetables to a plate to cool.

4   Season each fillet with salt and pepper.

5   Divide the vegetables between the fillets and roll them up. Place the rolled fish, seam side down, in the baking dish.

6   Pour the remaining ¼ cup of stock in the dish. Spoon the lemon juice over the fish. Dust with the paprika and sprinkle with the parsley. Bake 20 minutes until cooked through. Serve with Sautéed Sliced Potato and Onion (page 165).

SAUTÉED SLICED POTATO AND ONION

1 teaspoon olive oil

¼ cup thinly sliced onion

Pinch of salt

1 small Idaho potato, about 8 ounces, cut into thin, bite-size slices, about 1 cup

1 cup low-sodium chicken stock

Fresh ground black pepper to taste

2 teaspoons chopped fresh parsley

1   In an 8- to 10-inch nonstick skillet over medium heat, combine the oil, onion, and a pinch of salt and sauté, stirring for 2 to 3 minutes until lightly browned.

2   Add the potato and sauté 1 minute.

3   Pour in the chicken stock and simmer until almost dry, about 8 to 10 minutes. Season with salt and pepper. Stir in the parsley and serve.

PER SERVING:

262 calories	42 g protein	24 g total carbohydrates	8 g fiber	16 g net carbohydrates

Turkey Chili with Sautéed Potatoes

1 teaspoon olive oil

2 cloves garlic, crushed to a paste

12 ounces ground turkey

2 teaspoons chili powder

1 teaspoon ground cumin

1 teaspoon paprika

1 teaspoon onion powder

1 teaspoon Cajun seasoning

1/8 teaspoon cayenne pepper

1/2 cup tomato puree

1/4 cup water

1/2 teaspoon salt

1   Heat an 8- to 10-inch nonstick skillet over medium heat. Add the oil and garlic and sauté until golden. Add the turkey and cook 3 to 4 minutes, stirring frequently, until well browned.

2   Add the chili powder, cumin, paprika, onion powder, Cajun seasoning, and cayenne. Cook for 1 minute. Stir in the tomato puree, water, and salt. Simmer 3 to 4 minutes until thick. Serve over Sautéed Potatoes (page 167).

SAUTÉED POTATOES

1 teaspoon olive oil

1 Idaho potato, about 8 ounces, peeled and cut into ½-inch cubes

½ cup low-sodium chicken stock

Salt and fresh ground black pepper to taste

1   Heat an 8- to 10-inch nonstick skillet over medium heat. Add the oil and potato. Raise the heat to medium-high and sauté 3 to 5 minutes, stirring frequently, until the potato is well browned.

2   Add the chicken stock and lower the heat. Simmer covered for 10 to 12 minutes until the stock has been absorbed and the potatoes are tender. Season with salt and pepper.

PER SERVING:

284 calories	35 g protein	11.75 g total carbohydrates	1 g fiber	10.75 g net carbohydrates

Oatmeal-Almond–Crusted Flounder and Spicy Sautéed String Beans with Lemon Zest

SERVES 2

2 flounder fillets, 6 ounces each

½ teaspoon McCormick Lemon & Pepper Seasoning Salt

2 tablespoons low-sodium chicken stock or water

2 tablespoons quick-cooking oatmeal (1 minute, not instant)

3 tablespoons sliced almonds

½ teaspoon salt

¼ teaspoon fresh ground black pepper

2 teaspoons chopped fresh dill

2 slices lemon

1   Preheat the oven to 375°F. Lightly spray a 6 by 8-inch baking dish with Pam. Place the fish in the baking dish, pour chicken stock over fish, and dust with the lemon pepper seasoning.

2   Combine the oats, 1 tablespoon of the almonds, salt, pepper, and dill in a blender and grind to a meal.

3   Spread the meal over the fish and sprinkle with the remaining 2 tablespoons of almonds. Place a lemon slice on each fillet and spray with Pam.

4   Bake 20 minutes until cooked through. Serve with Spicy Sautéed String Beans with Lemon Zest (page 169).

SPICY SAUTÉED STRING BEANS WITH LEMON ZEST

2 cups haricots verts (slender French green beans) or regular green beans

1 teaspoon olive oil

1 clove garlic, finely chopped

Pinch of red pepper flakes

1 teaspoon finely grated lemon zest

1 teaspoon distilled white vinegar

Salt to taste

1   Steam the string beans in ½ inch of boiling water in a covered pan over high heat for 2 minutes until bright green but still quite crisp.

2   In an 8- to 10-inch nonstick skillet over medium heat, add the oil and garlic and sizzle until golden; do not brown. Add the string beans, red pepper flakes, and lemon zest. Sauté 2 minutes. Add the vinegar and cook 1 minute, season with salt, and serve.

PER SERVING:

256 calories	34.7 g protein	4.6 g total carbohydrates	1 g fiber	3.6 g net carbohydrates

Baked Chicken with Sautéed Escarole and Spicy Asian Rice Noodles

SERVES 2

12 ounces uncooked skinless boneless chicken breast, rinsed and dried

½ teaspoon salt

1 teaspoon McCormick Lemon & Pepper Seasoning Salt

Paprika to taste

1   Preheat the oven to 375°F. Lightly coat a 6 by 8-inch baking pan with Pam.

2   Place the chicken in the pan and sprinkle with the salt, lemon pepper seasoning, and paprika. Lightly spray the chicken with Pam and bake for 15 to 20 minutes until cooked through.

3   Serve with Sautéed Escarole and Spicy Asian Rice Noodles (page 171).

SAUTÉED ESCAROLE

2 teaspoons olive oil

1 teaspoon finely chopped garlic

1 medium head escarole, cored and rinsed

2 tablespoons low-sodium chicken stock

Salt and pepper to taste

1   Heat the oil in a 10- to 12-inch nonstick skillet over medium heat. Add the garlic and sauté 30 seconds until pale gold. Do not brown.

2   Add the escarole and chicken stock. Raise the heat and cook covered 3 to 5 minutes until wilted, then drain. Season with salt and pepper.

SPICY ASIAN RICE NOODLES

1 quart lightly salted water

2 ounces wide rice noodles

¼ teaspoon toasted sesame oil

½ teaspoon wheat-free tamari soy sauce

Pinch of McCormick Lemon & Pepper Seasoning Salt

2 to 3 drops Tabasco sauce

1   Bring the water to a boil in a medium saucepan. Add the noodles and cook for 5 minutes until tender. Stir occasionally to prevent sticking.

2   Drain well and transfer the noodles to a bowl. Toss with the remaining ingredients and serve immediately.

PER SERVING:

360 calories	45 g protein	38.5 g total carbohydrates	8 g fiber	30.5 g net carbohydrates

Grilled Mahimahi with Julienned Vegetables and Pineapple Salsa

SERVES 2

2 mahimahi fillets, about 6 ounces each, skin removed

Salt and fresh ground pepper to taste

1 teaspoon olive oil

1 cup julienned eggplant, from 1 small eggplant

1 cup julienned carrots, from 2 medium carrots

1 cup julienned red bell pepper, from 1 red bell pepper

2 tablespoons low-sodium chicken stock

1   Lightly season the fillets with salt and pepper.

2   Lightly spray a grill pan and place it over medium heat. Grill the fillets for 3 minutes per side until cooked through.

3   While the fish cooks, heat a 10- to 12-inch nonstick skillet over high heat. Add the oil, eggplant, carrots, and pepper. Season with salt and pepper and sauté for 2 minutes until lightly browned. Add the chicken stock, reduce the heat to low, and simmer covered for 2 to 3 minutes until the vegetables are crisp-tender.

4   Divide the vegetables between two plates and top each fillet with a spoonful of Pineapple Salsa (page 173).

PINEAPPLE SALSA

1 cup chopped fresh pineapple

2 tablespoons chopped fresh cilantro

2 to 3 drops Tabasco

Juice of ½ lime

¼ teaspoon Splenda (sugar-free sweetener)

Combine all the ingredients in a bowl. Serve spooned over the mahimahi as directed on page 172.

PER SERVING:

248 calories	37.4 g protein	20 g total carbohydrates	8 g fiber	12 g net carbohydrates

Stuffed Chicken with Portobello and Spinach, Sweet Peas and Carrots

SERVES 2

2 whole uncooked boneless skinless chicken breasts, about 6 ounces each

1 teaspoon dried basil

1 teaspoon dried thyme

1 teaspoon dried oregano

2 cloves garlic, crushed to a paste

½ teaspoon salt

¼ teaspoon fresh ground black pepper

1 large portobello mushroom cap, sliced

3 ounces prewashed packaged baby spinach, about 5 cups firmly packed

2 tablespoons low-sodium chicken stock

Fresh ground black pepper to taste

¼ teaspoon paprika

1   Preheat the oven to 375°F. Lightly spray a 6 by 8-inch baking pan with Pam.

2   Lay the chicken in the pan, smooth side down, and season with the basil, thyme, oregano, garlic, salt, and pepper.

3   Lightly spray a 10- to 12-inch nonstick skillet with Pam and place it over high heat. Sauté the portobello slices for 1 to 2 minutes until lightly browned. Add the spinach and chicken stock. Sauté 1 minute until the spinach wilts. Drain the spinach and discard any remaining cooking juice.

4   Divide the mushroom and spinach mixture between the chicken breasts in the baking pan. Roll up each breast and turn the smooth side up. Season them with salt and pepper and dust with paprika. Lightly spray the stuffed chicken breasts with Pam and bake for 20 to 25 minutes until cooked through. Serve with Sweet Peas and Carrots (page 175).

SWEET PEAS AND CARROTS

1 cup low-sodium chicken stock

½ cup finely diced carrot

½ cup frozen sweet peas

Salt and fresh ground black pepper to taste

1   Place a 1- to 2-quart saucepan over medium heat and add the stock. Add the carrot and simmer covered for 3 to 5 minutes until tender.

2   Add the peas and simmer covered for 2 minutes. Season with salt and pepper and serve.

PER SERVING:

305 calories	42 g protein	9.6 g total carbohydrates	2.25 g fiber	7.35 g net carbohydrates

Chicken Rollatini with Savory Mushroom Brown Rice

SERVES 2

2 whole uncooked boneless skinless chicken breasts, about 6 ounces each

½ teaspoon McCormick Lemon & Pepper Seasoning Salt

Salt and fresh ground black pepper to taste

8 slender spears asparagus, trimmed

¼ cup thinly sliced onion

2 ounces packaged baby spinach, about 4 cups firmly packed

2 tablespoons low-sodium chicken stock

1 clove garlic, crushed to a paste

¼ teaspoon paprika

1 recipe Savory Mushroom Brown Rice (page 95)

1   Preheat the oven to 375°F.

2   Lightly spray a 6 by 8-inch baking pan with Pam. Lay the chicken in the pan, smooth side down, and season with lemon pepper seasoning, salt, and pepper.

3   Steam the asparagus over ½ inch of boiling water in a covered pan for 2 minutes until tender. Drain and transfer to a plate to cool.

4   Lightly spray a medium skillet with Pam. Add the onion, garlic, and sauté over high heat for 1 to 2 minutes until lightly browned. Add the spinach and chicken stock. Sauté until the spinach wilts, about 1 to 2 minutes.

5   Divide the asparagus and spinach mixture between the chicken breasts in the pan. Roll up each breast and turn the smooth side up. Season them with salt and pepper and dust with paprika. Lightly spray the rollatini with Pam and bake for 20 to 25 minutes until cooked through. Serve with the Mushroom Brown Rice.

PER SERVING:

340 calories	49 g protein	33.6 g total carbohydrates	7.5 g fiber	26.1 g net carbohydrates

Chicken Rollatini with Roasted Peppers and Asparagus

Salt and fresh ground black pepper to taste

1 clove garlic, crushed to a paste

½ teaspoon dried basil

½ teaspoon dried oregano

1 teaspoon olive oil

2 whole uncooked boneless skinless chicken breasts, about 6 ounces each

8 slender spears asparagus, trimmed

1 roasted red pepper from a jar, sliced into strips

¼ teaspoon paprika

2 tablespoons low-sodium chicken stock or water

1 recipe Thyme-Roasted Potatoes (page 178)

1   Preheat the oven to 375°F.

2   Lightly spray a 6 by 8-inch baking pan with Pam.

3   In a small bowl combine the salt, pepper, garlic, basil, oregano, and olive oil. Place the chicken in the bowl and rub thoroughly with the spices. Transfer the chicken to the prepared pan smooth side down.

4   Steam the asparagus over ½ inch of boiling water in a covered pan for 2 minutes until tender. Drain and transfer to a plate to cool.

5   Divide the asparagus and pepper strips between the chicken breasts in the pan and roll to form neat packages. Turn the stuffed breasts smooth side up. Season with salt and pepper and dust with paprika. Add the chicken stock or water to the pan. Bake for 20 to 25 minutes until just cooked through. Serve with Thyme-Roasted Potatoes.

PER SERVING:

225 calories	42 g protein	11 g total carbohydrates	3 g fiber	8 g net carbohydrates

Sesame-Crusted Sea Scallops with Thyme-Roasted Potatoes and Sautéed Sugar Snap Peas

SERVES 2

8 large sea scallops (about 8 ounces)

Salt and fresh ground black pepper to taste

1 tablespoon sesame seeds

1 tablespoon fresh lemon juice

1. Place an 8- to 10-inch nonstick skillet over high heat.

2. Season the scallops with salt and pepper and toss with the sesame seeds.

3. When the pan is smoking hot, reduce the heat to medium and spray with Pam.

4. Add the scallops and sear for 2 minutes per side. Add the lemon juice and simmer 1 minute longer. Serve over Thyme-Roasted Potatoes (below) with Sautéed Sugar Snap Peas (page 179) on the side.

THYME-ROASTED POTATOES

SERVES 2

1 medium red potato, about 8 ounces total

½ teaspoon olive oil

½ teaspoons dried thyme

Salt and fresh ground black pepper to taste

1   Preheat the oven to 375°F.

2   Slice the potato into ¼-inch-thick rounds. Toss with the oil and thyme.

3   Season with salt and pepper. Spread the potatoes in a single layer on a non-stick baking sheet. Roast for 15 to 20 minutes until fork-tender.

SAUTÉED SUGAR SNAP PEAS

SERVES 2

1 cup sugar snap peas, strings removed

½ teaspoon olive oil

1 to 2 tablespoons water

Salt and fresh ground black pepper to taste

1   In a 6- to 8-inch sauté pan over medium heat, sauté the peas and oil, stirring occasionally, for 1 to 2 minutes.

2   Add 1 to 2 tablespoons of water and cover the pan.

3   Steam for 30 seconds until tender. Season with salt and pepper and serve.

PER SERVING:

193 calories	23 g protein	16 g total carbohydrates	1.5 g fiber	14.5 g net carbohydrates

Veal and Pepper Stew
à la Marinara
with Brown Rice

1 teaspoon olive oil

8 ounces boneless veal stew meat

1 clove garlic, crushed to a paste

Salt and fresh ground black pepper to taste

1 cup marinara sauce, no sugar added

1 cup water

1 red bell pepper, cored and sliced into ½-inch-wide strips

⅛ teaspoon dried oregano

2 tablespoons chopped fresh basil

1 cup cooked brown rice

1 tablespoon chopped fresh parsley

1   Preheat the oven to 300°F.

2   In a heavy 2-quart ovenproof saucepan or casserole over medium heat, add the oil, veal, and garlic. Sauté 5 to 7 minutes until the veal is well browned; season with salt and pepper.

3   Stir in the marinara sauce and water. Raise the heat to high and bring to a boil. Cover the pan and transfer to the oven. Bake for 1½ hours. Check occasionally and add more water if the veal appears dry.

4   Add the pepper, oregano, and basil. Return to the oven for 30 to 45 minutes until the veal is fork-tender. Season with salt and pepper. Serve over brown rice sprinkled with the chopped parsley.

PER SERVING:

365.9 calories	44 g protein	29 g total carbohydrates	7 g fiber	22 g net carbohydrates

STAYING ON TRACK: WHILE YOU'RE ON THE PLAN

On pages 13–16, I've given you some helpful tips on how to make sure you don't get caught without a healthy meal. But with our busy schedules, we all have days when we just don't have time to cook, or when we need to grab something on the run.

As with any lifestyle change, the first choice is obviously to stick to a meal that falls within the plan. If you can't, here are a few quick grabs that can keep your energy up and your sugar cravings away:

- Store-bought hummus spread on rice cakes or soy chips

- Peanut butter (sugar-free) on apple slices

- Turkey or beef jerky

- A handful of nuts (almonds or macadamia nuts are best)

- Soy nuts

- On the go, keep deli-roasted turkey and roast beef on hand. They are quick low-carb snacks and can be eaten in a pinch.

- An individual can of tuna fish is a simple, high-protein option that can be paired with a tossed salad for a quick meal.

- Kiss your George Foreman grill hello again! Grilling a 6-ounce chicken breast takes just 5 minutes! Pair it with two rice cakes and some broccoli spears for an on-the-go lunch.

- Rotisserie chickens can be found just about anywhere! They are delicious and protein-packed. Leave the skin at home!

In general, you'll want to look for foods that are high in protein. Legumes are a great choice because they not only contain protein, but fiber as well. Roasted soybeans are a great example. Many high-protein, high-fiber sports bars are readily available, which are also low in carbohydrates. Make sure to read the package carefully to be certain that your choice is a healthy one.

DINING OUT: A SIMPLE GUIDE TO MAKING GOOD CHOICES

Going out to eat is a favorite American pastime. Millions of us flock to restaurants every week and destroy our diets. Here is a short list of options to help those of us who are determined not to sabotage all of our hard work.

CHINESE: Bad news . . . many of our favorite dishes are fried and sugar-filled. To fight the bulge, order a steamed dish (most establishments nowadays have a diet menu) with sauce on the side; that way you can add only what you need. Eat only half the rice; a standard portion of steamed rice is double the amount you should eat.

JAPANESE: This can be a great place for the health conscious! Calorie and fat counts are lower in most foods; however, beware of the sodium. Ask the chef to prepare the meal for you with less (or no) salt, and beware of soy sauce; if you must, use it sparingly. Stay away from tempura, agemono, katsu, or any other breaded or fried dishes.

MEXICAN: Although typical Mexican ingredients such as corn, beans, and tomatoes, are healthy, these good foods often come smothered in high-fat, high-calorie cheeses and sour cream. If you can, skip the sauces altogether; the exception is salsa, which I recommend as a wonderful, low-calorie condiment. Order grilled meats with tomatillo sauce. Skip the tortilla shells, and even if you order guacamole, keep your hands off the chips!

ITALIAN: According to Denise Webb, a nutritional consultant and associate editor for the *Environmental Nutrition Newsletter: One plate of fettuccini Alfredo has as much saturated fat as 3 pints of Breyers Butter Almond ice cream!* There are plenty of meats and chicken dishes to enjoy, but opt for a red sauce, and stay away from Alfredo, carbonara, Parmigiana, or any cheeses. Most restaurants will accommodate a request to replace pasta with rice, which I recommend doing; eat half your portion and double up on the salad. My favorite dish is grilled shrimp over broccoli rabe; ask them to go very light on the oil. Some restaurants will even steam it for you.

Our society is so "bread-happy." It seems that no matter where we go out to eat, bread is on the table, or brought to it as soon as we're seated. Plan ahead and just say *"no"* to the bread basket. If it's not on the table, it will be much more difficult for you to load up on those extra empty calories!

If alcohol is part of your lifestyle, it's best to avoid it. If you must indulge, limit yourself to 1 serving and stay away from any juices or mixers with a lot of sugar. Clear liquors such as gin and vodka are naturally better than liqueurs and creamy concoctions.

CONDIMENTS

Condiments are widely used to add flavor to meals after they have been prepared. With so many different varieties on the market, I have composed a list of acceptable and unacceptable types. Typically, I do not use any for my personal consumption, as I have learned to love the natural taste of my foods. You can use these items prudently, however. Beware of hidden sugars and high-sodium contents.

Acceptable condiments

- hot sauce

- mustard

- lemon juice

- vinegar

- salsa

- pepper

- Mrs. Dash

- Low-sodium Molly McButter

- Cajun seasonings

The following condiments vary widely in acceptability. Check the labels for sugar content and use them sparingly.

- ketchup (Walden Farms makes a sugar-free ketchup)

- steak sauce

- barbecue sauce

Undesirable condiments

- all soy sauces (you can, however, use tamari soy sauce—a wheat-free alternative)

- teriyaki sauce

- Worcestershire sauce

- all fat-free condiments: sour cream, mayonnaise, salad dressings, etc.

Small amounts of salt are fine for seasoning foods, but refrain from using too much salt or salt-based seasonings.

FRUIT

The low-carb recipes in this book contain minimal fruit, as the sugar content is factored in. When beginning the plan, I usually recommend not eating additional fruit for the first two weeks, or at least until your sugar cravings diminish. As you embark on your new lifestyle, you will find that within the first week, your hunger will diminish. You will lose the cravings for "something sweet." If you find that you cannot do without it, choose your fruit carefully and try to avoid eating it in addition to a meal—you will want to space it out around 2 hours before or after. Following, you will see the carbohydrate content of most common fruits. When choosing, you'll want to stay at or around 15 grams of carbohydrates. The fruits in italics are higher than this recommended amount in their normal serving size, so you should avoid them or eat them in smaller amounts.

FRUIT	CARBOHYDRATE CONTENT (IN GRAMS)
Apple (½ medium)	10.5
Apricot—fresh (3 whole)	**11.7**
Avocado—California (½)	6.0
Avocado—Florida (½)	**13.5**
Banana—small	*23.7*
Blackberries—fresh (½ cup)	**9.2**
Blueberries—fresh (½ cup)	10.2
Boysenberries—fresh (½ cup)	**9.2**
Cantaloupe, chopped (½ cup)	7.4
Cantaloupe, medium (¼ section)	**11.6**
Cherries, sour—fresh (½ cup)	6.3
Cherries, sweet—fresh (½ cup)	**14.6**
Cranberries, raw, no sugar (½ cup)	6.0
Dates, chopped (½ cup)	*65.4*
Dates, fresh (3)	18.3
Figs, canned in water (½ cup)	**17.4**
Figs—fresh (1 small)	7.7
Fruit salad, canned in heavy syrup (½ cup)	*23.5*
Fruit salad, canned in juice (½ cup)	*16.3*
Grapefruit, fresh (½ cup)	9.5
Grapes, green seedless (½ cup)	14.2
Grapes, red seedless (½ cup)	**14.2**
Honeydew, chopped (½ cup)	7.8
Kiwifruit (1)	**11.3**
Kumquat (4)	12.5
Lychees, fresh (10 whole)	*15.9*
Mango, fresh (½ cup)	14.0
Orange (1)	*16.3*
Papaya, fresh (½ small)	7.5
Peach, canned in water (½ cup)	**7.5**

FRUIT	CARBOHYDRATE CONTENT (IN GRAMS)
Peach, fresh (1 small)	8.8
Pear, canned in water (½ cup)	9.5
Pear, fresh Bartlett (1 small)	25.1
Pear, fresh Bosc (1 small)	21.0
Persimmon (½ small)	15.6
Pineapple, canned in water (½ cup)	10.2
Pineapple, fresh chunks (½ cup)	9.6
Plum, fresh (1 small)	3.7
Pomegranate (½)	13.2
Prune, dried (4)	21.1
Raisins, golden (1 tablespoon)	8.2
Raisins, seedless (1 tablespoon)	8.1
Raspberries, fresh (½ cup)	7.1
Rhubarb, fresh (½ cup)	2.8
Strawberries, fresh (½ cup)	2.8
Tangerine (1)	7.8
Watermelon, chopped (½ cup)	5.5

SUGAR-FREE ARTIFICIAL SWEETENERS

In an effort to replace sugar, most of us turn to artificial sweeteners. Here is the skinny on some popular sugar replacements.

ASPARTAME—the blue stuff
Found in brands such as NutraSweet and Equal, aspartame is commonly found in diet sodas and soft drinks, or in the little blue packages to stir into coffee, tea, or on bowls of cereal. Usually 180 to 200 times sweeter than sugar, it contains about 4 calories per tablespoon. Lately, there has been a lot of controversy on this product and its safety. The food and drug administration has not, as of yet, required any warnings on the packaging.

SACCHARIN—the pink stuff
The subject of years of controversy, saccharin is currently sold with a label warning that it may cause cancer. Containing only ⅛ calorie per teaspoon, it is up to 300 times sweeter than sugar. This artificial sweetener is found in Sweet'N Low.

SUCRALOSE—the yellow stuff

Derived from natural sugars, this product is gaining popularity and can now be found in a variety of soft drinks and on most grocery shelves. Containing less than 1 calorie per teaspoon, sucralose can be up to 600 times sweeter than sugar and retains its sweetness when heated. Sucralose is found in the artificial sweetener Splenda. Because this product is the newest on the market, there have yet to be any warnings issued regarding its usage.

Eliminating sugar is essential in a low-carb diet and most of us will turn to artificial sweeteners to replace the sugar. I recommend eating mostly whole foods and meals that are free of chemicals, since we do not yet know the long-term effects of each artificial sweetener. In some recipes you will find I replace sugar with Splenda. Use your judgment, and find what is comfortable for you.

STAYING ON TRACK: BEYOND THE **5 SQUARE** MEAL MAKEOVER PLAN

Congratulations on your 5 squares 20-day makeover plan success. The journey, although it's undoubtedly become much easier for you, has really just begun. From here forward you embark on a lifelong path to better health and well-being. Thousands of individuals like you have successfully changed their eating habits and have not only gained confidence, but lost unwanted weight, inches, and body fat.

A few words that may help you on your way . . .

What do I do now? I thought you'd never ask. Now it is time to take the skills that you have learned and turn them into a way of life. You have realized that eating at least 5 meals a day has given you the energy of your youth. You have slept better, your appearance has changed, and your cravings for high-carb foods have diminished. Sugar has become an afterthought to you: Foods taste better and richer without any additives. You have become more organized, and you now plan your healthy selections well in advance so as not to be caught without good choices. You feel empowered and totally in control.

Take it to go! Most restaurants serve 2 to 4 times the amount of food you should eat in one sitting. If you are on the aggressive side, tell them to portion it the way *you* want it, and take the rest home for future meals. If not, eat a healthy amount, and ask for the leftovers to be wrapped up.

Get out of that chair! Active individuals are happier, thinner, and healthier. Take the stairs in lieu of the elevator. Park at the farthest end of the shopping mall. Play with your kids. Walk the dog. Vacuum, mow the lawn, accompany your kids to the bus stop or school yard. Chase your husband (or wife) around the bedroom.

Replace treats with treats! The thought of getting a manicure or buying a new article of clothing is far more appealing than eating a cookie. *Reward yourself*—you deserve it!

Make a fist! After completing the 20-day plan, you've probably become an expert at measuring portions. If you haven't already, learn to measure portions with your eye. Make a fist, a good way to measure a portion; 6 ounces of protein should not be much bigger than the average fist. Test it yourself on a scale if you are uncertain. Your starchy carbohydrate (potato, rice, etc.) should measure about half that. This skill will be important at all those business lunches, family gatherings, and other out-of-the-home events.

Add a salad! It is great to add a crunchy salad to your mealtime. Avoid dressings that contain sugar.

Take a second look! Refer back to the recipes. Try new combinations. If you get stuck or want to innovate, you can refer back to pages 13–16 and create your own meals according to the proper proportions of protein, starch, and carbohydrate.

If embarking on your own journey seems scary, then start it all over again! Begin at square 1—literally!

Last (but not least), enjoy your healthy life and make every day count! We would love to hear from you. Write us—nothing makes me happier than to hear of your success. Our e-mail address is info@my5squares.com.

Best of health and happy eating!

Monica Lynn

GLOSSARY

ADDITIVES (IN FOOD)— Food additives are substances intentionally added to either maintain shelf-life (freshness) or make foods more appealing.

ARTIFICIAL SWEETENERS— High-intensity sugar substitutes that include aspartame, saccharin, and sucralose.

ASIAN NOODLES— Some Asian noodles are wheat-based, but the majority are made from ingredients such as rice flour, buckwheat flour, or soybean starch. Although Asian egg noodles are wheat-based, a vast majority of other types can be found at Asian markets and are now gaining popularity in most health food stores. I strongly recommend that you look for the wheat-free varieties.

BARLEY— A wheat-free hearty grain used in dishes from cereals to breads and meal accompaniments.

BETA CAROTENE— Believed to be a powerful antioxidant, it is found in vegetables such as carrots, broccoli, squash, spinach, and sweet potatoes.

BROWN RICE— The entire rice grain with only the inedible outer husk removed. It is nutritious and higher in fiber than traditional white rice and has a nutty flavor and chewy texture.

BUCKWHEAT— This herb, which evolved from Russia, is usually thought of as a cereal or grain; however, the seeds from the plant are used to make buckwheat flour. When eaten as a whole food, it is derived from the hulled crushed kernels called buckwheat groats. It is high in fiber and recommended over wheat.

CALCIUM— A mineral vital for building and maintaining healthy bones and teeth. Calcium also provides for muscle contraction as well as proper clotting of blood. It is found not only in dairy products but in leafy green vegetables such as broccoli, spinach, and kale.

CALORIE— A standardized unit measuring the energy value of foods. Calories can be obtained from four sources: alcohol, carbohydrates, fats, and proteins.

CANADIAN BACON— Lean smoked meat taken from the tender eye of the loin in the middle of the back of the pig. Costing much more than traditional bacon, it is much leaner and precooked, therefore yielding more servings per pound.

CANOLA OIL— Expressed from rape seeds, its popularity is rising quickly in the United States because it is lower in saturated fat than any other oil. It also contains Omega-3 fatty acids, which have been shown to lower both cholesterol and triglycerides.

CARBOHYDRATE— A category of sugars, starches, fiber, and vegetables that the body breaks down into glucose, its primary source of energy. *Simple carbohydrates* are the sugars from glucose, fructose, sucrose, and lactose; they are absorbed very quickly into the body. *Complex carbohydrates* are most commonly found in whole grains and beans; they take longer to digest and usually provide more nutrients than simple carbohydrates.

EGG SUBSTITUTE— Commonly sold in cartons, this liquid is usually a blend of egg whites, food starch, corn oil, skim milk powder, tofu, and many different additives. It is lower in cholesterol; however, it is as high in sodium as a whole egg.

EGG WHITES— The clear substance left after removing the yolk from the egg. An excellent source of protein and riboflavin, it has no cholesterol.

FIBER— Dietary fiber is the portion of plant-related foods that cannot be entirely digested. It is therefore referred to as roughage. Fruits, beans, vegetables, and whole grains are all high-fiber plant-related foods.

GLUTEN— A grayish, elastic protein resembling chewing gum that is the result of wheat and other grains being made into flour. Most flours contain gluten in varying amounts, as it helps breads and other baked goods to rise.

JULIENNE— To cut foods into thin matchstick-like strips.

LACTOSE— Sometimes referred to as milk sugar, it occurs naturally in milk and is commonly used in baby formulas and candies.

MARINATE— The soaking of meat, fish, or vegetables to intensify the flavor of the food or in the case of meats, to tenderize.

MESCLUN— A mix of young, small salad greens commonly found in supermarkets and produce shops.

MILK FAT— Fatty particles in milk that are used to make cream and butter. The greater the milk fat content a food has, the richer and more caloric it is.

MOLASSES— The brownish liquid remaining from the refining process of sugarcane and sugar beets.

NONDAIRY CREAMER— The main function of this product is to lighten coffee and dilute the flavor. Nondairy creamer is made from coconut oil, palm or hydrogenated oil, sweeteners, and preservatives; it is high in saturated fat and is not recommended for those on low-cholesterol diets.

OATS— The most nutritious of cereals, the word in the literal term applies to a type of animal feed; however, we commonly know them as *oat groats*. These are oats that have been cleaned, toasted, hulled, and cleaned again. They can be cooked and served as a cereal or made into gluten-free flour.

ORGANIC FOODS— Foods that have been processed and grown without the use of chemicals of any sort—pesticide-free.

PINCH— A measuring term for a dry ingredient such as salt or pepper; the equivalent of 1/16 of a teaspoon.

POTATO FLOUR— Also called *potato starch*; a gluten-free flour made from potatoes, commonly used as a thickener and in some baked goods.

PROTEIN— Obtained from both animal and vegetable sources, it supplies energy and helps in repairing and building tissues.

RICE BRAN— The outer layer of a grain of rice, it is high in soluble fiber and has been proven effective in lowering cholesterol.

RICE FLOUR— Fine flour made from white rice. Rice flour is used mainly for baked goods.

RICE VINEGAR— Asian vinegar made from fermented rice.

SORBITOL— Found naturally in some fruits, this artificial sweetener is used in candies, gums, and other food products.

SOYBEAN— Lower in carbohydrates and higher in protein than any other bean, it is quite possibly the most economical source of protein in the world. A good source of iron, soy products are inexpensive and packed with nutrition.

SOY CHEESE— Cheese-like product made from soy milk. Soy cheese can be found in most health food stores and is growing in popularity.

SOY MILK— Iron-rich liquid made from pressing ground, cooked soybeans. Soy milk is higher in protein than cow's milk and is cholesterol-free.

SOY SAUCE— An Asian cooking staple, this dark salty sauce is made by fermenting soybeans and roasted wheat. In this book we replace soy sauce with wheat-free tamari soy sauce.

SPELT— An ancient cereal grain with a nutty flavor. It is easily digestible and higher in protein than wheat.

SUCROSE— Sugar obtained from sugarcane or sugar beets. It is still considered sugar, and should be avoided on a low-carbohydrate diet.

SUGAR— Almost 100 percent of this substance is pure carbohydrates. A cup of sugar in its various forms can contain anywhere from 700 to 900 calories per cup.

TAMARI— Similar to soy sauce, this thicker dark sauce is made from soybeans and is usually wheat-free.

WHEAT— A high-gluten cereal grain.

Some of the recipe ingredients are harder to find than others. Listed below are the websites that we use to locate or order products that fit into the 5 squares lifestyle:

www.Maplegrovefarms.com/sugar_free.html: For sugar-free maple syrup

www.Arrowheadmills.com: For wheat-free baking mixes and flours

www.waldenfarms.com: For all dressings mentioned in the book (sugar-free honey-Dijon, sun-dried tomato, Thousand Island, etc.) and for sugar-free marinara, ketchup, barbecue, and cocktail sauces

www.McCormick.com: For Lemon & Pepper Seasoning Salt and for Grill Mates Roasted Garlic Montreal Chicken Seasoning blend

www.organickingdom.com: For wheat-free tamari soy sauce

www.vtspecialtyfoods.org/members/vtbread.html: For spelt bread

www.vitasoy-usa.com: For Vitasoy products and links to Nasoya (Nayonaise)

FURTHER READING

To learn more about the effects of sugar on the body, an excellent resource is *Lick the Sugar Habit*, Nancy Appleton, Ph.D. Garden City, N.Y.: Avery Publishing Group, 1996.

The nutritional information was researched by using the following:

The Nutribase Nutrition Facts Desk Reference, 2d ed., New York: Avery/Penguin Putnam, Inc., 2001.

The Complete Book of Food Counts, Corinne T. Netzer. 6th ed. New York: Dell Publishing/Random House, 2003.